Sjögren's Syndrome

Editor

MICHAEL T. BRENNAN

ORAL AND MAXILLOFACIAL SURGERY CLINICS OF NORTH AMERICA

www.oralmaxsurgery.theclinics.com

Consulting Editor

RICHARD H. HAUG

February 2014 • Volume 26 • Number 1

ELSEVIER

1600 John F. Kennedy Boulevard ● Suite 1800 ● Philadelphia, Pennsylvania, 19103-2899

http://www.oralmaxsurgery.theclinics.com

ORAL AND MAXILLOFACIAL SURGERY CLINICS OF NORTH AMERICA Volume 26, Number 1
February 2014 ISSN 1042-3699, ISBN-13: 978-0323-26672-7

Editor: John Vassallo; j.vassallo@elsevier.com
Developmental Editor: Yonah Korngold

Oral and Maxillofacial Surgery Clinics of North America (ISSN 1042-3699) is published quarterly by Elsevier Inc., 360 Park Avenue South, New York, NY 10010-1710. Months of issue are February, May, August, and November. Business and Editorial Offices: 1600 John F. Kennedy Blvd., Suite 1800, Philadelphia, PA 19103-2899. Periodicals postage paid at New York, NY and additional mailing offices. Subscription prices are $385.00 per year for US individuals, $567.00 per year for US institutions, $175.00 per year for US students and residents, $455.00 per year for Canadian individuals, $680.00 per year for Canadian institutions, $520.00 per year for international individuals, $680.00 per year for international institutions and $235.00 per year for Canadian and foreign students/residents. To receive student/resident rate, orders must be accompanied by name or affiliated institution, date of term, and the *signature* of program/residency coordinator on institution letterhead. Orders will be billed at individual rate until proof of status is received. Foreign air speed delivery is included in all *Clinics* subscription prices. All prices are subject to change without notice. **POSTMASTER:** Send address changes to *Oral and Maxillofacial Surgery Clinics of North America,* Elsevier Periodicals Customer Service, 11830 Westline Industrial Drive, St. Louis, MO 63146. Tel: 1-800-654-2452 (U.S. and Canada); 314-447-8871 (outside U.S. and Canada). Fax: 314-447-8029. E-mail: journalscustomerservice-usa@elsevier.com (for print support); journalsonlinesupport-usa@elsevier.com (for online support).

Reprints. For copies of 100 or more, of articles in this publication, please contact the Commercial Reprints Department, Elsevier Inc., 360 Park Avenue South, New York, NY 10010-1710. Tel.: 212-633-3874; Fax: 212-633-3820; Email: reprints@elsevier.com.

Oral and Maxillofacial Surgery Clinics of North America is covered in *MEDLINE/PubMed* (*Index Medicus*), *Science Citation Index Expanded (SciSearch®)*, *Journal Citation Reports/Science Edition*, and *Current Contents®/Clinical Medicine*.

Printed and bound by CPI Group (UK) Ltd, Croydon, CR0 4YY

Transferred to digital print 2012

Contributors

CONSULTING EDITOR

RICHARD H. HAUG, DDS
Carolinas Center for Oral Health,
Charlotte, North Carolina

EDITOR

**MICHAEL T. BRENNAN, DDS, MHS,
FDS, RCSEd**
Professor and Director, Sjögren's Syndrome
and Salivary Disorders Center, Carolinas
Medical Center, Department of Oral Medicine,
Charlotte, North Carolina

AUTHORS

**MICHAEL T. BRENNAN, DDS, MHS,
FDS, RCSEd**
Professor and Director, Sjögren's Syndrome
and Salivary Disorders Center, Carolinas
Medical Center, Department of Oral Medicine,
Charlotte, North Carolina

STEVEN E. CARSONS, MD
Professor of Medicine, State University of
New York at Stony Brook School of Medicine,
Stony Brook; Chief, Division of Rheumatology,
Allergy, and Immunology, Winthrop University
Hospital, Mineola, New York

**KONSTANTINA DELLI, DDS, MSc,
Dr med dent**
Department of Oral and Maxillofacial
Surgery, University Medical Center Groningen,
University of Groningen, Groningen,
The Netherlands

ANDREA HERMAN, RDH, BS
Oral Medicine Dental Hygienist, Department
of Oral Medicine, Carolinas Center for Oral
Health, Charlotte, North Carolina

SABATINO IENOPOLI, DO
Division of Rheumatology, Allergy and
Immunology, Department of Medicine,

Winthrop University Hospital, Mineola; State
University of New York at Stony Brook School
of Medicine, Stony Brook, New York

SIRI BEIER JENSEN, DDS, PhD
Section of Oral Medicine, Clinical Oral
Physiology, Oral Pathology and Anatomy,
Department of Odontology, Faculty of
Health and Medical Sciences, University
of Copenhagen, Copenhagen, Denmark

MALIN V. JONSSON, DMD, PhD
Broegelmann Research Laboratory,
Department of Clinical Science, Haukeland
University Hospital; Section for Oral and
Maxillofacial Radiology, Department of
Clinical Dentistry, University of Bergen,
Bergen, Norway

RAFAEL MADERO-VISBAL, MD, FACS
Research Assistant, MD Anderson Cancer
Center, Orlando, Orlando, Florida

ZVONIMIR MILAS, MD, FACS
Director, Head and Neck Cancer Center,
Levine Cancer Institute; Associate Professor,
UNC School of Medicine, Charlotte Campus,
Charlotte, North Carolina

JOEL J. NAPEÑAS, DDS, FDS RCS(Ed)
Assistant Professor, Division of Oral Medicine
and Radiology, Schulich School of Medicine
and Dentistry, Western University, London,
Ontario, Canada; Department of Oral Medicine,
Carolinas Medical Center, Charlotte,
North Carolina

JENENE L. NOLL, RN, BSN
Clinical Care Coordinator, Department of
Oral Medicine, Sjögren's Syndrome and
Salivary Disorders Center, Carolinas
Medical Center, Charlotte, North Carolina

ANDRES PINTO, DMD, MPH, FDS RCSEd
Chairman, Department of Oral and
Maxillofacial Medicine and Diagnostic
Sciences, University Hospitals Case
Medical Center and Case Western Reserve
University School of Dental Medicine,
Cleveland, Ohio

TOVE R. REKSTEN, MPh, PhD
Broegelmann Research Laboratory,
Department of Clinical Science, Haukeland
University Hospital, University of Bergen,
Bergen, Norway

TANYA S. ROULEAU, DMD, FDS RCS(Ed)
Director, General Practice Residency
Program, Department of Oral Medicine,
Carolinas Medical Center, Charlotte,
North Carolina

VIDYA SANKAR, DMD, MHS, FDS RCSEd
Associate Professor, Director, Oral Medicine
Clinic, Dental School, University of Texas
Health Science Center San Antonio,
San Antonio, Texas

FRED K.L. SPIJKERVET, DMD, PhD
Professor and Chairman, Department of Oral
and Maxillofacial Surgery, University Medical
Center Groningen, University of Groningen,
Groningen, The Netherlands

STEVEN TAYLOR, MBA, BA
Chief Executive Officer, Sjögren's Syndrome
Foundation, Bethesda, Maryland

MICHAEL D. TURNER, DDS, MD, FACS
Director, New York Center for Salivary Gland
Diseases, Head and Neck Institute, Beth Israel
Medical Center, New York; Division Chief,
Oral and Maxillofacial, Jacobi Medical Center,
Bronx, New York

ARJAN VISSINK, DDS, MD, PhD
Professor, Department of Oral and
Maxillofacial Surgery, University Medical
Center Groningen, University of Groningen,
Groningen, The Netherlands

JASON J. WU, DO
Division of Rheumatology, Allergy and
Immunology, Department of Medicine,
Winthrop University Hospital, Mineola;
Nassau University Medical Center, East
Meadow, New York

Contents

Sjögren's syndrome may also cause mononuclear infiltration and immune complex deposition involving extraglandular sites producing several extraglandular manifestations (EGM). The prevalence of EGMs varies greatly depending on the particular manifestation. This article examines the ways that EGMs may present in patients with primary Sjögren's syndrome. The focus is on the more prevalent and significant EGMs including involvement of the nervous system, pulmonary manifestations, vasculitis associated with primary Sjögren's syndrome, and arthropathy.

Management of Extraglandular Manifestations of Primary Sjögren's Syndrome 101

Jason J. Wu and Steven E. Carsons

Primary Sjögren's syndrome can have multiple extra-glandular manifestations ranging from mild to severe. Treatment for extra-glandular manifestations is organ specific and therapies are targeted based on the primary organs involved. Preferred treatment options used for extra-glandular manifestations of Sjögren's syndrome are usually extrapolated from the physician's experience in treating similar manifestations in other autoimmune conditions such as rheumatoid arthritis and systemic lupus erythematous. The lack of immunomodulating disease modifying drugs in Sjögren's syndrome can be frustrating for patients dealing with extra-glandular manifestations, however recent advances in the field has made the future look promising for new therapeutic options.

Coping Strategies and Support Networks for Sjögren's Syndrome Patients 111

Andrea Herman, Steven Taylor, and Jenene Noll

Sjögren's syndrome is a chronic systemic autoimmune disease that can affect any organ system in the body. The most common symptoms are dryness of the mouth and eyes resulting from chronic inflammation and a progressive loss of secretory function. As with most individuals managing a chronic condition, patients with Sjögren's are on a multipronged path to disease and symptom management. Various coping strategies are presented in this article and the advantages and disadvantages discussed. Additionally, how a support group functions and practical guidance for the initiation of a Sjögren's support group are discussed.

Index 117

ORAL AND MAXILLOFACIAL SURGERY CLINICS OF NORTH AMERICA

RELATED INTEREST

Atlas of the Oral and Maxillofacial Surgery Clinics of North America
September 2013 (Vol. 21, No. 2)
Office Procedures for the Oral and Maxillofacial Surgeon
Stuart E. Lieblich, DMD, *Editor*

THE CLINICS ARE NOW AVAILABLE ONLINE!
Access your subscription at:
www.theclinics.com

Preface
Sjögren's Syndrome

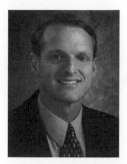

Michael T. Brennan, DDS, MHS, FDS, RCSEd
Editor

Sjögren's syndrome is a systemic autoimmune inflammatory condition impacting women more frequently than men (9:1) and is often diagnosed between the ages of 40 and 60, although it is not uncommon for symptoms to start much earlier than an official diagnosis. The most common symptoms of Sjögren's include dry mouth, dry eyes, and fatigue, although many other organ systems can be impacted in patients with this condition.

The field of Sjögren's has made significant advances in recent years, although much work is still needed to understand the many aspects of this condition. The overall goal of this issue of *Oral and Maxillofacial Surgery Clinics of North America* is to provide an up-to-date review by international experts of key topics vital to understanding this complex condition.

The articles in the current issue cover a wide range of topics, including the latest in the epidemiology and pathophysiology of Sjögren's; utilization and controversies of the different classification criterias currently used for Sjögren's, and considerations and techniques for salivary gland biopsies currently used to establish a Sjögren's diagnosis. Three articles present the oral signs and symptoms of Sjögren's and the evidence base for managing the oral sequelae of Sjögren's. Two articles explore the different salivary gland disease and the medical/surgical aspects for managing conditions, ranging from salivary gland infection to lymphoma. Additional articles provide the latest literature regarding the wide range of extraglandular manifestations of Sjögren's and the management strategies for these conditions. Finally, the last article explores patient coping strategies and the role of the Internet and support groups to assist with patients managing their chronic autoimmune condition.

The information presented in this issue provides the latest regarding the complex issues of Sjögren's, as well as points to the many research opportunities necessary to enhance our understanding of Sjögren's.

Michael T. Brennan, DDS, MHS, FDS, RCSEd
Sjögren's Syndrome and
Salivary Disorders Center
Department of Oral Medicine
Carolinas Medical Center
1000 Blythe Boulevard
Charlotte, NC 28232, USA

E-mail address:
Mike.Brennan@carolinashealthcare.org

http://dx.doi.org/10.1016/j.coms.2013.10.001
1042-3699/14/$ – see front matter

Sjögren's Syndrome
An Update on Epidemiology and Current Insights on Pathophysiology

Tove R. Reksten, MPh, PhD[a], Malin V. Jonsson, DMD, PhD[a,b],*

KEYWORDS

- Primary Sjögren's syndrome • pSS • Autoimmune diseases • Inflammatory disorder
- Epidemiology • Salivary glands • Pathogenesis

KEY POINTS

- Primary Sjögren's syndrome (pSS) is an autoimmune disease that affects 0.2% to 3.0% of the population.
- Nine of 10 patients with pSS are female.
- Primary SS is characterized by chronic inflammation of the exocrine glands, dryness symptoms, secretory dysfunction, and autoantibodies.
- Cytokines, chemokines, and survival factors attract and retain various subsets of chronic inflammatory cells in the target organ of pSS.
- Genetic studies indicate roles for certain cytokine genes and genetic factors regulating B-cell differentiation in the pathogenesis of pSS.
- NHL occurs in 4% to 5% of patients with pSS and is associated with certain risk factors.

INTRODUCTION

Sjögren's syndrome is an autoimmune rheumatic disease characterized by focal mononuclear cell infiltration of the salivary and lachrymal glands.[1] Primary Sjögren's syndrome (pSS) occurs alone, whereas secondary Sjögren's syndrome occurs in association with other autoimmune diseases, frequently rheumatoid arthritis (RA) and systemic lupus erythematosus (SLE).[2] Signs of systemic autoimmune disease with musculoskeletal, pulmonary, gastric, hematological, dermatologic, renal, and neurologic manifestations may also be evident in patients with SS.[1,3]

Common complaints are dryness of the mouth (xerostomia), and difficulties with talking, tasting, and swallowing.[4] Xerostomia is typically first noticed, as it becomes necessary to have chewing gum or lozenges on hand to stimulate saliva production, and by the urge to drink water during the night. Problems with speaking and eating due to reduced saliva secretion may ultimately lead to isolation of patients with the potential risk for depression and reduced quality of life, as well as severe problems linked to poor oral health.[5] Changes in secretion and composition of saliva, and higher dental caries activity have been suggested as potential markers to determine the autoimmune salivary gland dysfunction in pSS.[6]

Dry eyes (keratoconjunctivitis sicca) are often described as a sensation of grit or sand in the eyes, redness, itching, and photosensitivity. As with saliva, the tear flow and tear composition is altered in patients with pSS.[7] The dryness may also affect the airways, and reduced secretory capacity of sebaceous glands cause to be seen xerosis in up to 30% of patients with pSS.[8] Other cutaneous manifestations include erythemas, vasculitis, and dermatitis.

[a] Broegelmann Research Laboratory, Department of Clinical Science, University of Bergen, The Laboratory Building, 5th Floor, Haukeland University Hospital, Bergen N-5021, Norway; [b] Section for Oral and Maxillofacial Radiology, Department of Clinical Dentistry, University of Bergen, Årstadveien 19, Bergen N-5009, Norway
* Corresponding author.
E-mail address: Malin.Jonsson@iko.uib.no

Oral Maxillofacial Surg Clin N Am 26 (2014) 1–12
http://dx.doi.org/10.1016/j.coms.2013.09.002
1042-3699/14/$ – see front matter © 2014 Elsevier Inc. All rights reserved.

Tiredness and fatigue are other disabling complaints in pSS, contributing to work disability and depression,[9] and seem to remain mainly unchanged throughout the disease course.[10] Extraglandular manifestations, such as arthralgia and myalgia are reported by up to 75% and 45% of patients, respectively,[11,12] and Raynaud phenomenon is present in 10% to 15% of the patients, often preceding the onset of sicca symptoms.[13]

PREVALENCE AND INCIDENCE

SS has been suggested to affect 0.2% to 3.0% of the population.[14–16] It predominantly affects women between 40 and 60 years of age, with a 9:1 female:male ratio. Younger individuals and children may also be affected.[1] Most epidemiologic studies are based on hospital registries and research cohorts and then extrapolated to the general population. Regional differences are not extensively known.

There is no specific test for pSS, and a range of classification criteria have been applied over the years. Differences in items concerning dryness symptoms and autoimmune features have resulted in variations in prevalence, and depending on which criteria are used to diagnose the patients, the reported prevalence of pSS varies in different populations and with gender. In a Norwegian population-based study of 2 age groups, the prevalence was determined to be 0.22% in those 40 to 44 years old and 1.4% in those 71 to 74 years old.[17] In a local Norwegian population with 93% female patients, the prevalence was estimated at 0.05%.[18] This is in line with 0.09%[19] and 0.15%[16] in Greece, less than 0.1% to 0.4% in Great Britain,[15] and 0.17% in Brazil,[20] whereas a Turkish study including only women reported a prevalence of 0.72%.[21] A comparison of the recently introduced American College of Rheumatology (ACR) criteria for SS[22] to the American-European Concensus Group (AECG) criteria[2] showed 81% concordance in classification of pSS in 646 patients with sicca symptoms; 279 patients received the diagnosis by the AECG criteria and 268 by the ACR criteria. Regardless of classification, patients with pSS had similar gene expression profiles, which were different from healthy controls.[23]

The number of incidence studies of pSS is limited. A Slovenian study using the criteria from 1996[24] and an American study both suggested a yearly incidence of 3.9 per 100,000.[25,26] Odds ratio for SS was, in an Italian study, found to be 7.4 if the individual had a first-degree relative with autoimmune disease, and for women the risk was slightly higher in women who had given birth, with an odds ratio of 2.1.[27]

PATHOGENESIS OF SS
Histopathology of the Target Organ

The typical histopathological finding in labial minor salivary gland (MSG) biopsies is a progressive focal infiltration of mononuclear lymphoid cells.[28] A typical foci consists, per definition, of at least 50 mononuclear cells, such as lymphocytes, plasma cells, and macrophages, and is surrounded by otherwise normal-appearing glandular tissue (**Fig. 1**). The focus score, the number of foci per 4 mm^2 of MSG tissue, is associated with the presence of keratoconjunctivitis sicca and autoantibodies[29,30] and largely correlates with the reduced salivary secretion.[31] Despite lymphocytic infiltration and structural alterations within the MSGs, the remaining secretory acini seem to be functional and capable of secreting saliva.[6]

Another pattern of inflammation in labial MSG biopsies is chronic inflammation, characterized by scattered mononuclear cell infiltration without focal aggregates and accompanied by degenerative changes, such as acinar atrophy, ductal hyperplasia, fibrosis, and/or adipocyte infiltration.[32] Adipocytes are a possible source of chemokines[33]; resident adipocytes expressed CXCL12 in the MSGs of patients with pSS, possibly providing survival niches for long-lived plasma cells.

Studies have indicated a role for both the inflammatory cells and the salivary gland epithelium.[34] Salivary gland epithelial cells (SGEC) are themselves suggested to take part in the autoimmune inflammation seen in pSS MSG, expressing functional Toll-like receptors possibly inducing an innate immune response.[35] Furthermore, BAFF gene expression in SGEC was significantly

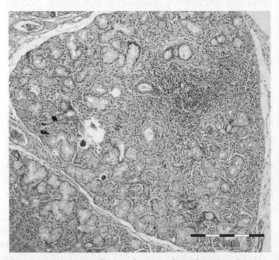

Fig. 1. Haematoxylin and eosin (H&E) stained minor salivary gland tissue section with focal mononuclear cell inflammation and surrounded by otherwise normal-appearing salivary gland tissue.

increased after both interferon (IFN)-α and IFN-γ stimulation,[36] with SGEC from patients with pSS significantly more susceptible to BAFF expression under stimulation with IFN-α than healthy controls. The same study found that SGEC from patients and healthy controls would secrete soluble BAFF after IFN-α and IFN-γ stimulation, adding a potential pathogenic role of SGEC in pSS. Costimulatory molecules are also shown to be expressed by epithelial cells in pSS, including CD80 and CD86 by ductal epithelial cells in patients with severe sialadenitis, as shown by immunohistochemical staining.[37,38] These cells may possibly be able to activate and stimulate T cells, as infiltrating CD28+ T cells were seen in close proximity to the CD80/CD8+ ductal cells.[38] SGECs do have the capacity to participate in the local autoimmune response, although how SGECs in pSS differ from SGECs in healthy controls remains to be seen.

Clinical Implications of Lymphoid Neogenesis

Lymphoid neogenesis in the form of germinal center (GC)-like structures; well-circumscribed inflammatory foci presenting with a dark and light zone,[39] has been described in the MSGs of 20% to 25% of patients with SS.[31,39–44] GC-like structures were characterized by B-cell and T-cell organization, increased levels of proliferating cells, follicular dendritic cell networks, activated endothelial cells, autoantibody producing cells and apoptotic events,[39,41,42] and B-cell expression of activation-induced cytidine deaminase (AICDA).[43] A certain clinical immunologic phenotype has been indicated in patients with GC-like structures (GC+)[31] and GC+ patients also exhibit aberrant cytokine profiles[32] and genetic traits.[45]

An association of GC development with increased risk of B-cell lymphomas, wherein formation of proliferating GCs were thought to contribute to malignant transformation and development of mucosa-associated lymphoid tissue (MALT) lymphoma has long been proposed.[46] Seven of 175 patients in a Swedish study went on to develop non-Hodgkin lymphoma (NHL) in a total of 1855 patient years at risk, with a median onset of 7 years following the initial diagnostic salivary gland biopsy. Six of the 7 patients had GC-like structures at diagnosis.[44] In a Greek study investigating major infiltrating cells in salivary gland infiltrates of various severity, 3 of 7 cases with lymphoma also presented with GC-like structures in the minor salivary glands.[40]

Local and Systemic Autoantibodies

Involvement of autoantibodies and cytokines are hallmarks of autoimmune disease. Autoantibodies

to the Ro/SSA and La/SSB proteins are included in the diagnostic criteria for pSS.[2,22] Antibodies to Ro/SSA are found in approximately 60% of patients, and antibodies to La/SSB in about 40%.[47] Systemic levels are reported to coincide with local autoantibody production.[39,48] Virtually all anti–La-positive patients are anti-Ro positive, and rheumatoid factor is present in 80% of patients.[49] Autoantibodies are also present in healthy individuals, but at lower titers and of different isotypes,[47] and age, but not disease manifestations, have been found to influence the presence of autoantibodies.[50] Recently, methods for detecting autoantibodies in saliva, in which levels are almost 4000-fold lower than in serum, have been developed, promising potential noninvasive diagnostic procedures.[51]

Antibodies directed against the Ro/La ribonucleoprotein complexes have been correlated with younger age,[29] more inflammation, and GC-like structures[31] and a higher prevalence of extraglandular manifestations, such as recurrent parotidomegaly, cutaneous vasculitis, Raynaud phenomenon, and renal involvement,[52] and arthralgia, arthritis, peripheral neuropathy, leukopenia, and thrombocytopenia.[53] Anti-Ro/SSA and anti-La/SSB are involved in development of neonatal lupus, characterized by skin rash, liver and hematological features, and congenital heart block.[54]

Other autoantibodies

Quite frequently, patients with pSS present with other autoantibodies than the hallmarking anti-Ro/SSA and anti-La/SSB. Indeed, in the ACR criteria, the presence of antinuclear antibodies (ANA) and rheumatoid factor (RF) may be sufficient for diagnosis.[22] Antimuscarinic 3 receptor (M3R) antibodies are present in sera of patients with pSS,[55] and are postulated to play a role in long-term loss of M3R function, giving a clue to understand the exocrinopathy in pSS,[56] being capable of damaging saliva production.[57] Anticentromere antibodies (ACA) were found in a small subpopulation of patients with pSS with a distinct disease phenotype.[58]

Various clinical associations have been described in relation to the diverse autoantibodies found in patients with SS (reviewed in Ref[59]).

Cytokines and Chemokines

Cytokines and chemokines attract T cells and monocytes, and also eosinophils, natural killer (NK) cells, and dendritic cells (DC). Cytokines play a pivotal role in the immune reaction, and patients with autoimmune diseases like pSS have a significantly different cytokine profile compared with healthy controls.[60] Elevated levels of cytokines and chemokines might be responsible for the increased recruitment and retention of lymphocytes to the MSGs and the ectopic GC-like structures found in the GC+ subgroup. Differences in cytokine profile in patients with and without myalgia are demonstrated,[61] and IFN-γ and eotaxin have been suggested as potential biomarkers for GC+ patients with pSS.[62] Type I interferons found in labial salivary gland biopsies, together with elevated serum levels of these cytokines, indicate a potential etiopathogenic mechanism for interferons.[63] The same study evaluated the capacity of pSS sera to induce IFN-α, and concluded that immune complexes of autoantibodies and RNA may be the inducers. IFN-α induces B cell differentiation and maintains Th1 cells,[64] and the type I IFN system has been suggested as a possible pathogenic mechanism in pSS.[65] A Th1 cytokine signature was seen in MSG samples from patients, although could not be correlated with disease severity.[66] Systemic levels of NCR3/NKp30, an NK cell specific activating receptor mediating cross-talk between NK cells and dendritic cells and type II IFN secretion, were increased in pSS and associated with INF-γ secretion, and accumulation of NK cells correlated with severity of exocrinopathy.[67]

Previous observations in which mRNA expression of IFN-γ only was detected in salivary glands of patients with pSS and not in healthy controls, whereas other cytokines, such as interleukin (IL)-6 and IL-10, were seen in both,[68] along with altered peripheral cytokine profiles,[69] led to the notion that T cells, and especially Th1 cells, are the main conductors of disease development and progression. In a Norwegian cohort of pSS, cytokines IL-17, IL-1RA, IL-15, macrophage inflammatory protein (MIP) 1α, MIP-1β, eotaxin, IFN-α, and IL-4 levels were significantly increased in GC+ patients. In addition, minor differences in cytokine levels were found when comparing age groups. Increased titers of Th17-associated cytokines, IL-17, IL-1β, and the IL-23 subunit IL-12p40, were speculated to indicate a higher activity of these cells in GC+ patients.[32]

Chemokines CXCL13 and CCL21 are produced by epithelial cells in relation to chronic inflammatory cells in MSGs from patients with SS.[33,39,70,71] Increased attraction, retention, and survival of inflammatory cells promote lymphoid structure formation (**Fig. 2**). In a murine model for SS, CXCL13 was associated with disease progression and blockade resulted in a slight reduction in glandular inflammation. In patients with SS, CXCL13 was elevated in serum and saliva, and saliva CXCL13 was associated with xerostomia.[72]

The presence of B-cell specific cytokines in pSS, such as upregulated B-cell activating factor

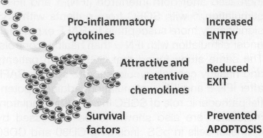

Pro-inflammatory cytokines — Increased ENTRY

Attractive and retentive chemokines — Reduced EXIT

Survival factors — Prevented APOPTOSIS

Fig. 2. Chronic inflammation in the MSGs of patients with Sjögren's syndrome may ultimately induce lymphoid neogenesis. Activated mononuclear cells such as T cells, B cells, and DCs are detected in the salivary glands as periductal chronic inflammatory cell infiltrates. Local production of cytokines and chemokines lead to attraction of T and B cells. Organized aggregates composed of T cells, B cells, FDC networks, activated endothelial cells, and plasma cells form GC-like structures. Long-term, inappropriate cytokine production and chemokine expression may lead to prolonged B-cell survival, possibly promoting neoplastic transformations in the target organ of SS.

(BAFF),[42,62] help explain the B-cell drive of the disease,[73] proving a possible target for treatment,[74] and contradicting the previous dogma that solely T cells are responsible for the abnormal cytokine production. Accumulation of chronic inflammatory cells in the target organ may be due to increased migration and/or a consequence of B-cell activation and differentiation in GC-like structures or by excess BAFF[75] favoring B-cell survival by antiapoptotic pathways, such as Bcl-2, a protein that mediates lymphocyte survival in a mitochondria-dependent way. Plasma cells marked for survival are increased in pSS and Bcl-2 seem to be induced by IL-6, which is associated with focus score.[33] In another study, peripheral blood monocytes produced significantly higher levels of sBAFF and IL-6 compared with monocytes from healthy controls, both following INF-γ stimulation and in absence of stimulation. Stimulation of monocytes by sBAFF induced IL-6 production, and expression of BAFF and transcription factors regulating IL-6 were increased in pSS monocytes.[76]

T Cells in pSS

Over the years, several studies have investigated the role of T cells in pSS. For one, T cells constitute up to 75% of the infiltrating cells, with 45% to 55% shown to be CD4+ cells and 15% to 35% being CD8+ cells, including transforming growth factor beta (TGF-β+) and Foxp3+ cells.[77] Furthermore, T-cell signature cytokines have important effector functions, including IFN-γ, IL-17, IL-21, and IL-4, and finally, T cells are important in the activation, maturation, and differentiation of autoantibody-producing plasma cells.

Cytotoxic T cells

The role of cytotoxic T cells (CTLs) in pSS pathogenesis has not been studied in detail, but novel autoantigen fragments after CTL-induced apoptosis have been reported in which unique structural autoantigen modifications have been suggested to occur during caspase-independent death pathways. Both caspase-3 and granzyme B cleaves La/SSB, and granzyme B cleaves the muscarinic 3 receptor (M3R), and if either is inhibited, altered cleavage may result in autoantigens. Indeed, antiapoptotic Bcl-2 members, inhibitors of endogenous caspase-3, are highly expressed in pSS epithelial cells.[78,79]

Autoreactive CTLs are seen in pSS targeting SS56.[80] SS56 is structurally related to Ro-52, and seronegative patients with pSS have been shown to have autoantibodies directed against SS56. SS56-specific CTLs were identified by IFN-γ enzyme-linked immunosorbent spot (ELISPOT) assay, and a later experiment did indeed show that SS56-specific CTLs from patients with pSS were capable of lysing $SS56_{55-64}$ loaded T cells.[81]

NKT cells

NKT cells are found in only limited amounts among circulating lymphocytes, and there is just one reported case of extranodal NKT-cell lymphoma in pSS.[82] Other findings with regard to NKT cells are contradicting, with reports of elevated levels of NKT cells in peripheral blood and in particular in patients with extraglandular manifestations,[83] and reports of reduced levels as compared with healthy controls.[84] The latter study postulated that this could be due to abnormality of NKT cells, with nonresponding patients (50%) presenting with cells that would not expand in the presence of APC from responders, and possibly due to overstimulation, as the responders did expand in vitro in spite of low numbers in vivo.

Follicular helper T cells

Recently, evidence of follicular helper T (Tfh) cells in pSS has emerged. Peripheral CD4+CXCR5+CCR6+ cells are found in increased amounts in pSS, and these levels are positively correlated with ESSDAI, immunoglobulin, Ro/SSA, and La/SSB.[85] Th17 subsets of CD4+CXCR5+ T cells may differentiate into Tfh and provide cognate help to antigen-specific B cells, which again may lead to differentiation into autoantibody-producing plasma cells. A higher frequency of this subset may also be a disease activity biomarker. Szabo and colleagues[86] found that the elevated ratios of Tfh cells could be attributed to the presence of extraglandular manifestations, and were further positively correlated with T-cell activation markers and negatively correlated with IgG and IgM memory B-cell populations.

Th17 cells

Th17 cells are the third subset of T helper cells.[87] Evidence that IL-17 mediates inflammatory autoimmune diseases is accumulating, with mice models describing Th17 and/or IL-17 involvement in RA,[88] psoriasis,[89,90] and diabetes.[91] Curiously, so far the IL-17 gene has not been reported as a susceptibility gene in autoimmune disease.[92]

Evidence of systemic involvement of Th17 in pSS is scarce, although elevated serum levels of Th17-associated cytokines in pSS have been reported.[32,93] Local minor salivary gland IL-17 expression has been verified by several groups,[93–95] but reported distribution patterns vary greatly, possibly due to specificity of immunostaining.[96]

A recent article rejected the suggestion that IL-17 is directly involved in B-cell antibody production in vivo.[97] Nonetheless, Th17 cells enhance B-cell proliferation, at least in mice,[98] and one might speculate whether one of the other Th17-associated cytokines, like IL-21, provide the Th17 help. IL-21R$^{-/-}$ mice have defective immunoglobulin production, and disorganized GC formation,[99] and IL-21 produced by Th17 cells may play a role in formation of the GC-like structures seen in some minor salivary gland tissue samples from patients with pSS, indicated by increased levels of Th17-associated cytokines in serum of GC+ patients.[32]

Aicda upregulation in GC B cells is associated with development of pathogenic autoantibodies in BXD2 mice, and activated CD4+ T cells are central regulators of autoreactive B cells.[100] The association of T cells to B cells in GCs was abrogated by IL-17 blocking agents,[101] and the same study showed that the absence of IL-17 resulted in a smaller GC response but also an altered follicular:marginal zone ratio of B cells. If IL-17 is crucial for the formation and stabilization of ectopic GCs, IL-17–positive staining in the GC-like structures in pSS minor salivary gland tissue would be expected, but has thus far not been reported.

The Treg/Th17 balance

The absolute ratio of Tregs in pSS peripheral blood (PB) and the MSGs is disputed. Although most findings point toward a lower ratio of CD4+ CD25^{high} cells in PB compared with healthy controls,[102,103] there were, however, no significant differences in the suppressive abilities of the cells from patients and healthy controls. On the other hand, Foxp3$^+$ cells seemed to correlate with inflammation grade in the MSG.[104,105]

The reciprocal relationship with Th17 cells is in a fine balance crucial for immune homeostasis. Two important cytokines, namely TGF-β and IL-6, are involved in the differentiation of these cells and the maintenance of the balance, and a skewed production of TGF-β and IL-6 is seen in MSG epithelial cells in pSS.[106] Increased IL-6 production seen in the MSG may explain the imbalance in regulation of Th17, fostering a pathogenic environment. Furthermore, Tregs represent a type of cells controlling and suppressing improper immune reactions, sustaining tolerance in the periphery. One might postulate that reduced levels of Tregs in pSS opens up for autoimmunity and breach of tolerance, whereas others postulate that there is a certain pool of Tregs, and with autoimmune inflammation in exocrine glands, they migrate from the periphery. The observation of fewer Treg cells in advanced than in mild salivary gland infiltrates support a view that DC-derived TGF-β may induce FoxP3 in naïve T cells and switch T-cell differentiation toward Th17 in the presence of IL-6.[107,108]

Genetics

A hereditary link was early suggested in SS, and, indeed, 35% of patients with pSS have relatives with other autoimmune diseases.[109] Susceptibility genes to SS are found in HLA-B8,[110] the tumor necrosis factor (TNF) system,[111] and in components of the type I IFN system.[112] Genetic polymorphisms in the promoter of NCR3/NKp30 were associated with reduced gene transcription and function, and seemed to have a protective role in pSS.[67]

Genetic association studies in pSS have thus far mainly been candidate gene studies, in which known gene associations in other autoimmune diseases have formed the basis. Susceptibility genes have been identified in several genes involved in B-cell differentiation, including EBF1, BLK, and TNFSF4,[113] although these SNPs showed no association to the presence of Ro/La autoantibodies. Another study reported genetic associations of TGF-β and TNF-α gene polymorphisms to the presence of anti-La antibodies rather than to the disease.[114] In a recent genome-wide association study (GWAS) of patients with pSS, IRF5, STAT4, and BLK, associations were confirmed and novel associations near IL12A, CXCR5, and TNIP1 established.[115]

Further proposals of genetic implications for the pSS etiology and autoantibody expression are the CTLA4 haplotypes, which are also possibly protective against development of Raynaud phenomenon.[116] The functional consequences of these genetic polymorphisms remain to be elucidated.

Nevertheless, disease susceptibility has been associated with HLA alleles, and Arnett and colleagues[117] demonstrated an association with HLA-DQ and strong autoantibody response in pSS. Some cytokine genes are shown or suggested to be associated with pSS and/or anti-Ro/SSA and/or anti-La/SSB, including the TNF-α and IL-10 genes,[114,118] a SNP in the Il2–Il21 region,[119] and Il6.[120] We examined possible associations of cytokine genes to the presence of GC-like structures in patients with pSS, and found that one SNP in Ccl11 (eotaxin) and one SNP in the Ccl7–Ccl11 region were associated with GC status.[45] This greatly supports our initial findings in which GC+ patients had elevated serum levels of CCL11, and also supports the conclusions from a discriminant function analysis suggesting CCL11 as 1 of 3 key discriminant biomarkers for GC+.[62] The CCL11 allele variant seen in GC+ patients seems to be protective, although patients have higher CCL11 serum levels than GC− patients. Interestingly, this is a phenomenon also observed in a congenic experimental autoimmune encephalomyelitis rat strain,[121] where CCL11 apparently is involved in a signaling pathway not related to eosinophil recruitment.[122]

RISK AND PREDICTION OF LYMPHOMA

Although mortality is not significantly increased in pSS compared with the general population,[123] a well-documented and severe complication is the progression to B-cell lymphoma.[124–126] The association between pSS and lymphoma has been studied over the past 50 years. At first the risk was overestimated due to a selected patient material,[125] whereas more recent population-based studies in Scandinavia indicate a 9-fold to 16-fold increase in risk[127,128] with NHL of the MALT type occurring in 4% to 5% of patients with pSS.[46] Several subtypes of NHL are associated with pSS, the most common being MALT lymphoma and diffuse large B-cell lymphoma (DLBCL), and a 28 times increased risk of MALT lymphoma and 11 times increased risk of DLBCL was determined.[129] In comparison with other autoimmune chronic inflammatory diseases, the risk for NHL in pSS is higher than in SLE and RA.[130] Patients with SS and chronic Helicobacter pylori infection are at increased risk for developing lymphomas, possibly related to prolonged lymphocytic activation in the target organ(s) of these patients.[131,132]

Recent suggestions for lymphoma prediction in SS include CD4 lympocytopenia[127] and GC-like structures in MSG biopsies.[44] Established predictors for lymphoma development in SS are recurrent or permanent swelling of major salivary glands, lymphadenopathy, cryoglobulinemia, splenomegaly, low complement levels of C4 and C3, lymphopenia, skin vasculitis or palpable purpura, M-component in serum or urine, peripheral neuropathy, glomerulonephritis, and elevated beta2-microglobulin (reviewed in Jonsson and colleagues[133]). Individuals with several risk factors or overlapping autoimmune diseases most likely have an increased risk of pSS-associated lymphoma.[134,135] Other suggested risk factors for lymphoma may be male gender[136] and duration of disease.[127,137]

In summary, pSS can have manifestations ranging from mild to severe, including significant oral and ocular symptoms, disabling fatigue, reduced quality of life, and, for some patients, an increased risk of developing lymphoma.

REFERENCES

1. Jonsson R, Bowman SJ, Gordon TP. Sjögren's syndrome. In: Koopman WJ, editor. Arthritis and allied conditions. 15th edition. Philadelphia: Lippincott WIlliams & Wilkins; 2005. p. 1681–705.

2. Vitali C, Bombardieri S, Jonsson R, et al. Classification criteria for Sjögren's syndrome: a revised version of the European criteria proposed by the American-European Consensus Group. Ann Rheum Dis 2002;61(6):554–8.

3. Manthorpe R, Jacobsson LT, Kirtava Z, et al. Epidemiology of Sjögren's syndrome, especially its primary form. Ann Med Interne (Paris) 1998;149(1): 7–11.

4. Jonsson MV, Delaleu N, Marthinussen MC, et al. Oral and dental manifestations of Sjögren's syndrome: current approaches to diagnostics and therapy. In: Fox RI, Fox C, editors. Sjögren's syndrome: pathogenesis and therapy. New York, Dordrecht (The Netherlands), Heidelberg (Germany), London: Springer; 2011. p. 221–42.

5. Brosky ME. The role of saliva in oral health: strategies for prevention and management of xerostomia. J Support Oncol 2007;5(5):215–25.

6. Pedersen AM, Bardow A, Nauntofte B. Salivary changes and dental caries as potential oral markers of autoimmune salivary gland dysfunction in primary Sjögren's syndrome. BMC Clin Pathol 2005;5(1):4.

7. Bjerrum KB. Tear fluid analysis in patients with primary Sjögren's syndrome using lectin probes. A comparative study of patients with primary Sjögren's syndrome, patients with other immune inflammatory connective tissue diseases and controls. Acta Ophthalmol Scand 1999;77(1):1–8.

8. Bernacchi E, Amato L, Parodi A, et al. Sjögren's syndrome: a retrospective review of the cutaneous features of 93 patients by the Italian Group of Immunodermatology. Clin Exp Rheumatol 2004; 22(1):55–62.

9. Barendregt PJ, Visser MR, Smets EM, et al. Fatigue in primary Sjögren's syndrome. Ann Rheum Dis 1998;57(5):291–5.

10. Haldorsen K, Bjelland I, Bolstad AI, et al. A five-year prospective study of fatigue in primary Sjögren's syndrome. Arthritis Res Ther 2011; 13(5):R167.

11. Haga HJ, Peen E. A study of the arthritis pattern in primary Sjögren's syndrome. Clin Exp Rheumatol 2007;25(1):88–91.

12. Lindvall B, Bengtsson A, Ernerudh J, et al. Subclinical myositis is common in primary Sjögren's syndrome and is not related to muscle pain. J Rheumatol 2002;29(4):717–25.

13. Garcia-Carrasco M, Siso A, Ramos-Casals M, et al. Raynaud's phenomenon in primary Sjögren's syndrome. Prevalence and clinical characteristics in a series of 320 patients. J Rheumatol 2002;29(4): 726–30.

14. Birlik M, Akar S, Gurler O, et al. Prevalence of primary Sjögren's syndrome in Turkey: a population-based epidemiological study. Int J Clin Pract 2009;63(6):954–61.

15. Bowman SJ, Ibrahim GH, Holmes G, et al. Estimating the prevalence among Caucasian women of primary Sjögren's syndrome in two general practices in Birmingham, UK. Scand J Rheumatol 2004; 33(1):39–43.

16. Trontzas PI, Andrianakos AA. Sjögren's syndrome: a population based study of prevalence in Greece. The ESORDIG study. Ann Rheum Dis 2005;64(8): 1240–1.

17. Haugen AJ, Peen E, Hulten B, et al. Estimation of the prevalence of primary Sjögren's syndrome in two age-different community-based populations using two sets of classification criteria: the Hordaland Health Study. Scand J Rheumatol 2008; 37(1):30–4.

18. Gøransson LG, Haldorsen K, Brun JG, et al. The point prevalence of clinically relevant primary Sjögren's syndrome in two Norwegian counties. Scand J Rheumatol 2011;40(3):221–4.

19. Alamanos Y, Tsifetaki N, Voulgari PV, et al. Epidemiology of primary Sjögren's syndrome in north-west Greece, 1982-2003. Rheumatology 2006;45(2): 187–91.

20. Valim V, Zandonade E, Pereira AM, et al. Primary Sjögren's syndrome prevalence in a major metropolitan area in Brazil. Rev Bras Reumatol 2013; 53(1):24–34.

21. Kabasakal Y, Kitapcioglu G, Turk T, et al. The prevalence of Sjögren's syndrome in adult women. Scand J Rheumatol 2006;35(5):379–83.

22. Shiboski SC, Shiboski CH, Criswell LA, et al. American College of Rheumatology classification criteria for Sjögren's syndrome: a data-driven, expert consensus approach in the Sjögren's International Collaborative Clinical Alliance Cohort. Arthritis Care Res 2012;64(4):475–87.

23. Rasmussen A, Ice JA, Li H, et al. Comparison of the American-European Consensus Group Sjögren's syndrome classification criteria to newly proposed American College of Rheumatology criteria in a large, carefully characterized sicca cohort. Ann Rheum Dis. [E-pub ahead of print].

24. Vitali C, Bombardieri S, Moutsopoulos HM, et al. Assessment of the European classification criteria for Sjögren's syndrome in a series of clinically defined cases: results of a prospective multicentre study. The European Study Group on Diagnostic Criteria for Sjögren's Syndrome. Ann Rheum Dis 1996;55(2):116–21.

25. Plesivcnik Novljan M, Rozman B, Hocevar A, et al. Incidence of primary Sjögren's syndrome in Slovenia. Ann Rheum Dis 2004;63(7):874–6.

26. Pillemer SR, Matteson EL, Jacobsson LT, et al. Incidence of physician-diagnosed primary Sjögren syndrome in residents of Olmsted County, Minnesota. Mayo Clin Proc 2001;76(6):593–9.

27. Priori R, Medda E, Conti F, et al. Risk factors for Sjögren's syndrome: a case-control study. Clin Exp Rheumatol 2007;25(3):378–84.

28. Jonsson R, Kroneld U, Backman K, et al. Progression of sialadenitis in Sjögren's syndrome. Br J Rheumatol 1993;32(7):578–81.

29. Atkinson JC, Travis WD, Slocum L, et al. Serum anti-SS-B/La and IgA rheumatoid factor are markers of salivary gland disease activity in primary Sjögren's syndrome. Arthritis Rheum 1992; 35(11):1368–72.

30. Daniels TE, Whitcher JP. Association of patterns of labial salivary gland inflammation with keratoconjunctivitis sicca. Analysis of 618 patients with suspected Sjögren's syndrome. Arthritis Rheum 1994;37(6):869–77.

31. Jonsson MV, Skarstein K, Jonsson R, et al. Serological implications of germinal center-like structures in primary Sjögren's syndrome. J Rheumatol 2007;34(10):2044–9.

32. Reksten TR, Jonsson MV, Szyszko EA, et al. Cytokine and autoantibody profiling related to histopathological features in primary Sjögren's syndrome. Rheumatology 2009;48(9):1102–6.

33. Szyszko EA, Brokstad KA, Øijordsbakken G, et al. Salivary glands of primary Sjögren's syndrome patients express factors vital for plasma cell survival. Arthritis Res Ther 2011;13(1):R2.

34. Manoussakis MN, Kapsogeorgou EK. The role of intrinsic epithelial activation in the pathogenesis of Sjögren's syndrome. J Autoimmun 2010;35(3): 219–24.

35. Spachidou MP, Bourazopoulou E, Maratheftis CI, et al. Expression of functional Toll-like receptors by salivary gland epithelial cells: increased mRNA expression in cells derived from patients with primary Sjögren's syndrome. Clin Exp Immunol 2007;147(3):497–503.

36. Ittah M, Miceli-Richard C, Eric Gottenberg J, et al. B cell-activating factor of the tumor necrosis factor family (BAFF) is expressed under stimulation by interferon in salivary gland epithelial cells in primary Sjögren's syndrome. Arthritis Res Ther 2006;8(2):R51.

37. Manoussakis MN, Dimitriou ID, Kapsogeorgou EK, et al. Expression of B7 costimulatory molecules by salivary gland epithelial cells in patients with Sjögren's syndrome. Arthritis Rheum 1999;42(2): 229–39.

38. Matsumura R, Umemiya K, Goto T, et al. Glandular and extraglandular expression of costimulatory molecules in patients with Sjögren's syndrome. Ann Rheum Dis 2001;60(5):473–82.

39. Salomonsson S, Jonsson MV, Skarstein K, et al. Cellular basis of ectopic germinal center formation and autoantibody production in the target organ of patients with Sjögren's syndrome. Arthritis Rheum 2003;48(11):3187–201.

40. Christodoulou MI, Kapsogeorgou EK, Moutsopoulos HM. Characteristics of the minor salivary gland infiltrates in Sjögren's syndrome. J Autoimmun 2010;34(4):400–7.

41. Jonsson MV, Skarstein K. Follicular dendritic cells confirm lymphoid organization in the minor salivary glands of primary Sjögren's syndrome. J Oral Pathol Med 2008;37(9):515–21.

42. Jonsson MV, Szodoray P, Jellestad S, et al. Association between circulating levels of the novel TNF family members APRIL and BAFF and lymphoid organization in primary Sjögren's syndrome. J Clin Immunol 2005;25(3):189–201.

43. Le Pottier L, Devauchelle V, Fautrel A, et al. Ectopic germinal centers are rare in Sjögren's syndrome salivary glands and do not exclude autoreactive B cells. J Immunol 2009;182(6):3540–7.

44. Theander E, Vasaitis L, Baecklund E, et al. Lymphoid organisation in labial salivary gland biopsies is a possible predictor for the development of malignant lymphoma in primary Sjögren's syndrome. Ann Rheum Dis 2011;70(8):1363–8.

45. Reksten TR, Johnsen SJ, Jonsson MV, et al. Genetic associations to germinal centre formation in primary Sjögren's syndrome. Ann Rheum Dis 2013. [Epub ahead of print].

46. Voulgarelis M, Dafni UG, Isenberg DA, et al. Malignant lymphoma in primary Sjögren's syndrome: a

multicenter, retrospective, clinical study by the European Concerted Action on Sjögren's Syndrome. Arthritis Rheum 1999;42(8):1765–72.

47. Garberg H, Jonsson R, Brokstad KA. The serological pattern of autoantibodies to the Ro52, Ro60, and La48 autoantigens in primary Sjögren's syndrome patients and healthy controls. Scand J Rheumatol 2005;34(1):49–55.

48. Salomonsson S, Wahren-Herlenius M. Local production of Ro/SSA and La/SSB autoantibodies in the target organ coincides with high levels of circulating antibodies in sera of patients with Sjögren's syndrome. Scand J Rheumatol 2003; 32(2):79–82.

49. Elkon KB, Gharavi AE, Hughes GR, et al. Autoantibodies in the sicca syndrome (primary Sjögren's syndrome). Ann Rheum Dis 1984;43(2):243–5.

50. Haga HJ, Jonsson R. The influence of age on disease manifestations and serological characteristics in primary Sjögren's syndrome. Scand J Rheumatol 1999;28(4):227–32.

51. Ching KH, Burbelo PD, Gonzalez-Begne M, et al. Salivary anti-Ro60 and anti-Ro52 antibody profiles to diagnose Sjögren's syndrome. J Dent Res 2011;90(4):445–9.

52. Martel C, Gondran G, Launay D, et al. Active immunological profile is associated with systemic Sjögren's syndrome. J Clin Immunol 2011;31(5): 840–7.

53. Ramos-Casals M, Solans R, Rosas J, et al. Primary Sjögren syndrome in Spain: clinical and immunologic expression in 1010 patients. Medicine 2008; 87(4):210–9.

54. Buyon JP. Neonatal lupus. Curr Opin Rheumatol 1996;8(5):485–90.

55. Marczinovits I, Kovacs L, Gyorgy A, et al. A peptide of human muscarinic acetylcholine receptor 3 is antigenic in primary Sjögren's syndrome. J Autoimmun 2005;24(1):47–54.

56. Jin M, Hwang SM, Davies AJ, et al. Autoantibodies in primary Sjögren's syndrome patients induce internalization of muscarinic type 3 receptors. Biochim Biophys Acta 2012;1822(2):161–7.

57. Dawson LJ, Stanbury J, Venn N, et al. Antimuscarinic antibodies in primary Sjögren's syndrome reversibly inhibit the mechanism of fluid secretion by human submandibular salivary acinar cells. Arthritis Rheum 2006;54(4):1165–73.

58. Bournia VK, Diamanti KD, Vlachoyiannopoulos PG, et al. Anticentromere antibody positive Sjögren's syndrome: a retrospective descriptive analysis. Arthritis Res Ther 2010;12(2):R47.

59. Bournia VK, Vlachoyiannopoulos PG. Subgroups of Sjögren syndrome patients according to serological profiles. J Autoimmun 2012;39(1–2):15–26.

60. Szodoray P, Alex P, Brun JG, et al. Circulating cytokines in primary Sjögren's syndrome determined by a multiplex cytokine array system. Scand J Immunol 2004;59(6):592–9.

61. Eriksson P, Andersson C, Ekerfelt C, et al. Sjögren's syndrome with myalgia is associated with subnormal secretion of cytokines by peripheral blood mononuclear cells. J Rheumatol 2004;31(4):729–35.

62. Szodoray P, Alex P, Jonsson MV, et al. Distinct profiles of Sjögren's syndrome patients with ectopic salivary gland germinal centers revealed by serum cytokines and BAFF. Clin Immunol 2005;117(2): 168–76.

63. Båve U, Nordmark G, Lövgren T, et al. Activation of the type I interferon system in primary Sjögren's syndrome: a possible etiopathogenic mechanism. Arthritis Rheum 2005;52(4):1185–95.

64. Theofilopoulos AN, Baccala R, Beutler B, et al. Type I interferons (alpha/beta) in immunity and autoimmunity. Annu Rev Immunol 2005;23:307–36.

65. Akdis M, Palomares O, van de Veen W, et al. TH17 and TH22 cells: a confusion of antimicrobial response with tissue inflammation versus protection. J Allergy Clin Immunol 2012;129(6): 1438–49.

66. Kolkowski EC, Reth P, Pelusa F, et al. Th1 predominance and perforin expression in minor salivary glands from patients with primary Sjögren's syndrome. J Autoimmun 1999;13(1):155–62.

67. Rusakiewicz S, Nocturne G, Lazure T, et al. NCR3/NKp30 contributes to pathogenesis in primary Sjögren's syndrome. Sci Transl Med 2013;5(195): 195ra96.

68. Sun D, Emmert-Buck MR, Fox PC. Differential cytokine mRNA expression in human labial minor salivary glands in primary Sjögren's syndrome. Autoimmunity 1998;28(3):125–37.

69. Hagiwara E, Pando J, Ishigatsubo Y, et al. Altered frequency of type 1 cytokine secreting cells in the peripheral blood of patients with primary Sjögren's syndrome. J Rheumatol 1998;25(1):89–93.

70. Salomonsson S, Larsson P, Tengner P, et al. Expression of the B cell-attracting chemokine CXCL13 in the target organ and autoantibody production in ectopic lymphoid tissue in the chronic inflammatory disease Sjögren's syndrome. Scand J Immunol 2002;55(4):336–42.

71. Xanthou G, Polihronis M, Tzioufas AG, et al. "Lymphoid" chemokine messenger RNA expression by epithelial cells in the chronic inflammatory lesion of the salivary glands of Sjögren's syndrome patients: possible participation in lymphoid structure formation. Arthritis Rheum 2001;44(2):408–18.

72. Kramer JM, Klimatcheva E, Rothstein TL. CXCL13 is elevated in Sjögren's syndrome in mice and humans and is implicated in disease pathogenesis. J Leukoc Biol 2013. [Epub ahead of print].

73. Cornec D, Devauchelle-Pensec V, Tobon GJ, et al. B cells in Sjögren's syndrome: from pathophysiology

to diagnosis and treatment. J Autoimmun 2012; 39(3):161–7.

74. Abdulahad WH, Kroese FG, Vissink A, et al. Immune regulation and B-cell depletion therapy in patients with primary Sjögren's syndrome. J Autoimmun 2012;39(1–2):103–11.

75. Mackay F, Browning JL. BAFF: a fundamental survival factor for B cells. Nat Rev Immunol 2002; 2(7):465–75.

76. Yoshimoto K, Tanaka M, Kojima M, et al. Regulatory mechanisms for the production of BAFF and IL-6 are impaired in monocytes of patients of primary Sjögren's syndrome. Arthritis Res Ther 2011; 13(5):R170.

77. Katsifis GE, Moutsopoulos NM, Wahl SM. T lymphocytes in Sjögren's syndrome: contributors to and regulators of pathophysiology. Clin Rev Allergy Immunol 2007;32(3):252–64.

78. Ayukawa K, Taniguchi S, Masumoto J, et al. La autoantigen is cleaved in the COOH terminus and loses the nuclear localization signal during apoptosis. J Biol Chem 2000;275(44):34465–70.

79. Rosen A, Casciola-Rosen L. Altered autoantigen structure in Sjögren's syndrome: implications for the pathogenesis of autoimmune tissue damage. Crit Rev Oral Biol Med 2004;15(3):156–64.

80. Billaut-Mulot O, Cocude C, Kolesnitchenko V, et al. SS-56, a novel cellular target of autoantibody responses in Sjögren syndrome and systemic lupus erythematosus. J Clin Invest 2001;108(6):861–9.

81. Baek Sorensen R, Faurschou M, Troelsen L, et al. Melanoma inhibitor of apoptosis protein (ML-IAP) specific cytotoxic T lymphocytes cross-react with an epitope from the auto-antigen SS56. J Invest Dermatol 2009;129(8):1992–9.

82. Yan B, Liu Y, Hu D, et al. A rare case of extranasal NK/T cell lymphoma presenting as autoimmune rheumatic manifestations associated with Sjögren's syndrome. Ann Hematol 2010;89(4):423–4.

83. Szodoray P, Papp G, Horvath IF, et al. Cells with regulatory function of the innate and adaptive immune system in primary Sjögren's syndrome. Clin Exp Immunol 2009;157(3):343–9.

84. Kojo S, Adachi Y, Keino H, et al. Dysfunction of T cell receptor AV24AJ18+, BV11+ double-negative regulatory natural killer T cells in autoimmune diseases. Arthritis Rheum 2001;44(5):1127–38.

85. Li XY, Wu ZB, Ding J, et al. Role of the frequency of blood CD4(+) CXCR5(+) CCR6(+) T cells in autoimmunity in patients with Sjögren's syndrome. Biochem Biophys Res Commun 2012;422(2):238–44.

86. Szabo K, Papp G, Barath S, et al. Follicular helper T cells may play an important role in the severity of primary Sjögren's syndrome. Clin Immunol 2013; 147(2):95–104.

87. Park H, Li Z, Yang XO, et al. A distinct lineage of CD4 T cells regulates tissue inflammation by producing interleukin 17. Nat Immunol 2005; 6(11):1133–41.

88. Nakae S, Nambu A, Sudo K, et al. Suppression of immune induction of collagen-induced arthritis in IL-17-deficient mice. J Immunol 2003;171(11): 6173–7.

89. Nakajima K, Kanda T, Takaishi M, et al. Distinct roles of IL-23 and IL-17 in the development of psoriasis-like lesions in a mouse model. J Immunol 2011; 186(7):4481–9.

90. Nakajima K, Kanda T, Takaishi M, et al. Correction: distinct roles of IL-23 and IL-17 in the development of psoriasis-like lesions in a mouse model. J Immunol 2011;187(11):6157–8.

91. Emamaullee JA, Davis J, Merani S, et al. Inhibition of Th17 cells regulates autoimmune diabetes in NOD mice. Diabetes 2009;58(6):1302–11.

92. Ghoreschi K, Laurence A, Yang XP, et al. T helper 17 cell heterogeneity and pathogenicity in autoimmune disease. Trends Immunol 2011;32(9):395–401.

93. Katsifis GE, Rekka S, Moutsopoulos NM, et al. Systemic and local interleukin-17 and linked cytokines associated with Sjögren's syndrome immunopathogenesis. Am J Pathol 2009;175(3): 1167–77.

94. Mieliauskaite D, Dumalakiene I, Rugiene R, et al. Expression of IL-17, IL-23 and their receptors in minor salivary glands of patients with primary Sjögren's syndrome. Clin Dev Immunol 2012; 2012:187258.

95. Sakai A, Sugawara Y, Kuroishi T, et al. Identification of IL-18 and Th17 cells in salivary glands of patients with Sjögren's syndrome, and amplification of IL-17-mediated secretion of inflammatory cytokines from salivary gland cells by IL-18. J Immunol 2008;181(4):2898–906.

96. Yapici U, Roelofs JJ, Florquin S. The importance of testing anti-IL-17 antibodies from different suppliers. Am J Transplant 2012;12(2):504–5 [author reply: 6].

97. Shibui A, Shimura E, Nambu A, et al. Th17 cell-derived IL-17 is dispensable for B cell antibody production. Cytokine 2012;59(1):108–14.

98. Mitsdoerffer M, Lee Y, Jager A, et al. Proinflammatory T helper type 17 cells are effective B-cell helpers. Proc Natl Acad Sci U S A 2010;107(32): 14292–7.

99. Ozaki K, Spolski R, Feng CG, et al. A critical role for IL-21 in regulating immunoglobulin production. Science 2002;298(5598):1630–4.

100. Hsu HC, Wu Y, Yang P, et al. Overexpression of activation-induced cytidine deaminase in B cells is associated with production of highly pathogenic autoantibodies. J Immunol 2007;178(8): 5357–65.

101. Hsu HC, Yang P, Wang J, et al. Interleukin 17-producing T helper cells and interleukin 17 orchestrate

autoreactive germinal center development in autoimmune BXD2 mice. Nat Immunol 2008;9(2):166–75.

102. Li X, Li X, Qian L, et al. T regulatory cells are markedly diminished in diseased salivary glands of patients with primary Sjögren's syndrome. J Rheumatol 2007;34(12):2438–45.

103. Liu MF, Lin LH, Weng CT, et al. Decreased CD4+CD25+bright T cells in peripheral blood of patients with primary Sjögren's syndrome. Lupus 2008;17(1):34–9.

104. Christodoulou MI, Kapsogeorgou EK, Moutsopoulos NM, et al. Foxp3+ T-regulatory cells in Sjögren's syndrome: correlation with the grade of the autoimmune lesion and certain adverse prognostic factors. Am J Pathol 2008;173(5):1389–96.

105. Sarigul M, Yazisiz V, Bassorgun CI, et al. The numbers of Foxp3 + Treg cells are positively correlated with higher grade of infiltration at the salivary glands in primary Sjögren's syndrome. Lupus 2010;19(2):138–45.

106. Kawanami T, Sawaki T, Sakai T, et al. Skewed production of IL-6 and TGFbeta by cultured salivary gland epithelial cells from patients with Sjögren's syndrome. PLoS One 2012;7(10):e45689.

107. Romagnani S. Human Th17 cells. Arthritis Res Ther 2008;10(2):206.

108. Youinou P, Pers JO. Disturbance of cytokine networks in Sjögren's syndrome. Arthritis Res Ther 2011;13(4):227.

109. Reveille JD, Wilson RW, Provost TT, et al. Primary Sjögren's syndrome and other autoimmune diseases in families. Prevalence and immunogenetic studies in six kindreds. Ann Intern Med 1984; 101(6):748–56.

110. Fye KH, Terasaki PI, Moutsopoulos H, et al. Association of Sjögren's syndrome with HLA-B8. Arthritis Rheum 1976;19(5):883–6.

111. Bolstad AI, Le Hellard S, Kristjansdottir G, et al. Association between genetic variants in the tumour necrosis factor/lymphotoxin alpha/lymphotoxin beta locus and primary Sjögren's syndrome in Scandinavian samples. Ann Rheum Dis 2012; 71(6):981–8.

112. Nordmark G, Kristjansdottir G, Theander E, et al. Additive effects of the major risk alleles of IRF5 and STAT4 in primary Sjögren's syndrome. Genes Immun 2009;10(1):68–76.

113. Nordmark G, Kristjansdottir G, Theander E, et al. Association of EBF1, FAM167A(C8orf13)-BLK and TNFSF4 gene variants with primary Sjögren's syndrome. Genes Immun 2011;12(2):100–9.

114. Gottenberg JE, Busson M, Loiseau P, et al. Association of transforming growth factor beta1 and tumor necrosis factor alpha polymorphisms with anti-SSB/La antibody secretion in patients with primary Sjögren's syndrome. Arthritis Rheum 2004; 50(2):570–80.

115. Lessard CJ, Li H, Adrianto I, et al. Identification of multiple genetic variants associated with Sjögren's syndrome involved in both the innate and adaptive immune responses. Nature genetics, in press, the paper is accepted for publication but not e-pub yet; hence in press.

116. Downie-Doyle S, Bayat N, Rischmueller M, et al. Influence of CTLA4 haplotypes on susceptibility and some extraglandular manifestations in primary Sjögren's syndrome. Arthritis Rheum 2006;54(8): 2434–40.

117. Arnett FC, Bias WB, Reveille JD. Genetic studies in Sjögren's syndrome and systemic lupus erythematosus. J Autoimmun 1989;2(4):403–13.

118. Hulkkonen J, Pertovaara M, Antonen J, et al. Genetic association between interleukin-10 promoter region polymorphisms and primary Sjögren's syndrome. Arthritis Rheum 2001;44(1):176–9.

119. Maiti AK, Kim-Howard X, Viswanathan P, et al. Confirmation of an association between rs6822844 at the Il2-Il21 region and multiple autoimmune diseases: evidence of a general susceptibility locus. Arthritis Rheum 2010;62(2):323–9.

120. Hulkkonen J, Pertovaara M, Antonen J, et al. Elevated interleukin-6 plasma levels are regulated by the promoter region polymorphism of the IL6 gene in primary Sjögren's syndrome and correlate with the clinical manifestations of the disease. Rheumatology 2001;40(6):656–61.

121. Öckinger J, Stridh P, Boyoon AD, et al. Genetic variants of CC chemokine genes in experimental autoimmune encephalomyelitis, multiple sclerosis and rheumatoid arthritis. Genes Immun 2010;11(2): 142–54.

122. Adzemovic MZ, Ockinger J, Zeitelhofer M, et al. Expression of Ccl11 associates with immune response modulation and protection against neuroinflammation in rats. PLoS One 2012;7(7): e39794.

123. Theander E, Manthorpe R, Jacobsson LT. Mortality and causes of death in primary Sjögren's syndrome: a prospective cohort study. Arthritis Rheum 2004;50(4):1262–9.

124. Anderson LG, Talal N. The spectrum of benign to malignant lymphoproliferation in Sjögren's syndrome. Clin Exp Immunol 1972;10(2): 199–221.

125. Kassan SS, Thomas TL, Moutsopoulos HM, et al. Increased risk of lymphoma in sicca syndrome. Ann Intern Med 1978;89(6):888–92.

126. Zulman J, Jaffe R, Talal N. Evidence that the malignant lymphoma of Sjögren's syndrome is a monoclonal B-cell neoplasm. N Engl J Med 1978; 299(22):1215–20.

127. Theander E, Henriksson G, Ljungberg O, et al. Lymphoma and other malignancies in primary Sjögren's syndrome: a cohort study on cancer

incidence and lymphoma predictors. Ann Rheum Dis 2006;65(6):796–803.

128. Johnsen SJ, Brun JG, Goransson LG, et al. Risk of non-Hodgkin's lymphoma in primary Sjögren's syndrome: a population-based study. Arthritis Care Res 2013;65(5):816–21.

129. Smedby KE, Hjalgrim H, Askling J, et al. Autoimmune and chronic inflammatory disorders and risk of non-Hodgkin lymphoma by subtype. J Natl Cancer Inst 2006;98(1):51–60.

130. Zintzaras E, Voulgarelis M, Moutsopoulos HM. The risk of lymphoma development in autoimmune diseases: a meta-analysis. Arch Intern Med 2005; 165(20):2337–44.

131. Raderer M, Osterreicher C, Machold K, et al. Impaired response of gastric MALT-lymphoma to *Helicobacter pylori* eradication in patients with autoimmune disease. Ann Oncol 2001;12(7): 937–9.

132. Streubel B, Huber D, Wohrer S, et al. Frequency of chromosomal aberrations involving MALT1 in mucosa-associated lymphoid tissue lymphoma in

patients with Sjögren's syndrome. Clin Cancer Res 2004;10(2):476–80.

133. Jonsson MV, Theander E, Jonsson R. Predictors for the development of non-Hodgkin lymphoma in primary Sjögren's syndrome. Presse Med 2012;41(9 Pt 2):e511–6.

134. Baimpa E, Dahabreh IJ, Voulgarelis M, et al. Hematologic manifestations and predictors of lymphoma development in primary Sjögren syndrome: clinical and pathophysiologic aspects. Medicine 2009; 88(5):284–93.

135. Zhang W, Feng S, Yan S, et al. Incidence of malignancy in primary Sjögren's syndrome in a Chinese cohort. Rheumatology 2010;49(3):571–7.

136. Ansell P, Simpson J, Lightfoot T, et al. Non-Hodgkin lymphoma and autoimmunity: does gender matter? Int J Cancer 2011;129(2):460–6.

137. Ioannidis JP, Vassiliou VA, Moutsopoulos HM. Long-term risk of mortality and lymphoproliferative disease and predictive classification of primary Sjögren's syndrome. Arthritis Rheum 2002;46(3): 741–7.

Diagnosis of Sjögren's Syndrome
American-European and the American College of Rheumatology Classification Criteria

Vidya Sankar, DMD, MHS, FDS RCSEd[a],*,
Jenene L. Noll, RN, BSN[b],
Michael T. Brennan, DDS, MHS, FDS RCSEd[b]

KEYWORDS

- Sjögren's syndrome • Diagnosis • Classification

KEY POINTS

- The terms diagnostic criteria and classification criteria for Sjögren's syndrome (SS) are frequently used interchangeably, although they represent different concepts; therefore, the differences are highlighted.
- Advances in the understanding of SS create the need for refinement of classification criteria.
- The major differences between and the strengths and weaknesses of the American European Consensus Group Criteria and the American College of Rheumatology (ACR) criteria for SS are addressed.
- Application of the more stringent ACR classification criteria in clinical practice may have an effect on reported prevalence of the disease.

INTRODUCTION

Sjögren's syndrome (SS) is a chronic, systemic autoimmune disorder with multiple organ system involvement, which lacks 1 single objective diagnostic gold standard, making diagnosis challenging. This situation is also true in other rheumatic diseases, such as systemic lupus erythematosus (SLE) and rheumatoid arthritis (RA). Each of these diseases has its own unique combination of clinical and laboratory manifestations, which are relied on when making a diagnosis. The clinician's judgment is the closest thing there is to a gold standard for diagnosis.

Classification criteria are used as a formalized approach to studying the course and management of rheumatic diseases and provide a conceptual base for measuring future improvements in clinical care. They usually focus on clinical objectives to improve clinical research activities.[1] They are dynamic and continually evolve, as our understanding of the disease increases. Diagnosis differs from classification criteria in that the latter attempts to categorize a more homogeneous population in an attempt to better assess response to treatments.

Since 1965, there have been 11 sets of classification criteria for SS.[2–12] Past classification criteria contain a combination of subjective and objective findings in 3 areas of specialty practice: rheumatology, ophthalmology, and oral medicine. Criteria

[a] Oral Medicine Clinic, Dental School, University of Texas Health Science Center San Antonio, 7703 Floyd Curl Drive, MC 7914, San Antonio, TX 78229, USA; [b] Sjögren's Syndrome and Salivary Disorders Center, Carolinas Medical Center, Department of Oral Medicine, 1000 Blythe Boulevard, Charlotte, NC 28203, USA
* Corresponding author.
E-mail address: sankarv@uthscsa.edu

Oral Maxillofacial Surg Clin N Am 26 (2014) 13–22
http://dx.doi.org/10.1016/j.coms.2013.09.001

oralmaxsurgery.theclinics.com

sets generally include the presence of serologic markers, objective oral and ocular findings assessing either function or changes in gland architecture or degree of damage, and subjective oral and ocular complaints.

Criteria sets have assessed glandular changes by the presence of focal lymphocytic infiltration or focus score (FS). This pathologic process occurs within the lacrimal glands, all 4 of the major salivary glands as well as the labial minor salivary glands (LSGs). Biopsy of the labial minor salivary gland is a less invasive procedure compared with biopsy of one of the major salivary glands or the lacrimal glands and is therefore the procedure of choice. One limitation associated with the LSG biopsy is that the sensitivity and specificity of this test vary widely (63%–93% and 61%–100%, respectively).[13] To complicate matters, the prevalence of focal lymphocytic infiltration in postmortem LSG studies ranges from 0% to 22.4% in males and 0% to 35.7% in females.[14] In addition, recent studies have shown that there are significant discrepancies in the evaluation of LSG biopsies among different pathologists, different specialties, and different specialty centers.[15,16] For this reason, classification criteria sets varied in what was considered a positive FS, ranging from an FS of more than 1 to 1 or more. Other objective tests of salivary gland function include salivary flow rates, scintigraphy, and sialography. These tests are associated with a variety of limitations, which are covered in more detail later.

Autoantibodies are another common component of classification criterion. Anti-Ro/SSA and anti-La/SSB antibodies are among the most frequently detected autoantibodies against extractable nuclear antigens associated with SS. Problematically, SSA has also been associated with SLE, systemic sclerosis, polymyositis, primary biliary cirrhosis, dermatomyositis, mixed connective tissue disease (CTD), and RA. The pathologic role of these antibodies is still poorly understood. Higher titers of SSA and SSB are associated with greater incidence of extraglandular manifestations of SS such as purpura, leukopenia, and lymphopenia.[17] Other less specific markers of inflammation such as IgG, antinuclear antibody (ANA), erythrocyte sedimentation rate, and rheumatoid factor (RF) have been included in past criteria.

Several ocular tests have been proposed for use in the classification of SS. Tests include tear breakup time, Schirmer tests with and without anesthesia, clearance tests, corneal esthesiometry, corneal and conjunctival staining with differing scoring and staining methods, and imprint cytology. These tests assess the ability of the lacrimal glands to function, the integrity of the tear film layers, or damage or deficits of the ocular surface.

Most of the previous classification criteria sets also included the presence of subjective symptoms of oral and ocular dryness in addition to these objective measures. The most commonly used symptom assessment criteria involve a positive response to at least 1 of the following 3 questions related to ocular symptoms: "Have you had daily, persistent, troublesome dry eyes for more than 3 months?"; "Do you have a recurrent sensation of sand or gravel in the eyes?"; and "Do you use tear substitutes more than 3 times a day?" Assessment of oral symptoms involves a positive response to at least 1 of the following: "Have you had a daily feeling of dry mouth for more than 3 months?"; "Have you had recurrently or persistently swollen salivary glands as an adult?"; and "Do you frequently drink liquids to aid in swallowing dry food?" The problem with assessing subjective complaints when determining SS classification is that dry eye and dry mouth symptoms are common and nonspecific.

According to the Dry Eye Workshop 2007 report, prevalence of dry eye ranges from 5% to 30% in people aged 50 years and older.[18] The prevalence of dry eye syndrome in the United States is estimated to be 3.2 million women and 1.7 million men, for a total of 4.9 million patients 50 years and older.[19] Prevalence estimates of xerostomia fluctuate depending on the population being studied but have been reported as high as 24.8%.[20]

Classification criteria are intended to provide a formalized approach to studying course and management of rheumatic disease, as well as a measure of improvement in clinical care. Understanding the purposes of specific criteria sets and the differences between different criteria categories is crucial for understanding the rheumatic disease literature and for the design and conduct of clinical and epidemiologic investigations.[1] In this article, the similarities and differences between the American-European Consensus Group Criteria (AECG)[9] and the newly proposed American College of Rheumatology (ACR) classification criteria for SS are described.[21] The clinical implications of switching to the ACR classification criteria from the AECG are also explored.

AECG CRITERIA

The AECG criteria (**Box 1**) published in 2002 were developed after criticisms were raised about the European Study Group on Classification Criteria (ESGCC) for SS,[8] which were developed and validated between 1989 and 1996 and were subject to certain bias based on a combination of ocular

---

Box 1
AECG criteria for SS

I. Ocular symptoms: a positive response to at least 1 of the following questions:

   1. Have you had daily, persistent, troublesome dry eyes for more than 3 months?

   2. Do you have a recurrent sensation of sand or gravel in the eyes?

   3. Do you use tear substitutes more than 3 times a day?

II. Oral symptoms: a positive response to at least 1 of the following questions:

   1. Have you had a daily feeling of dry mouth for more than 3 months?

   2. Have you had recurrently or persistently swollen salivary glands as an adult?

   3. Do you frequently drink liquids to aid in swallowing dry food?

III. Ocular signs, that is, objective evidence of ocular involvement defined as a positive result for at least 1 of the following 2 tests:

   1. Schirmer I test, performed without anesthesia (<5 mm in 5 minutes)

   2. Rose bengal score or other ocular dye score (>4 according to van Bijsterveld scoring system)

IV. Histopathology: in minor salivary glands (obtained through normal-appearing mucosa), focal lymphocytic sialoadenitis, evaluated by an expert histopathologist, with an FS greater than 1, defined as several lymphocytic foci (which are adjacent to normal-appearing mucous acini and contain >50 lymphocytes) per 4 mm^2 of glandular tissue

V. Salivary gland involvement: objective evidence of salivary gland involvement defined by a positive result for at least 1 of the following diagnostic tests:

   1. Unstimulated whole salivary flow (<1.5 mL in 15 minutes)

   2. Parotid sialography showing the presence of diffuse sialectasias (punctate, cavitary, or destructive pattern), without evidence of obstruction in the major ducts according to the scoring system of Rubin and Holt[36]

   3. Salivary scintigraphy showing reduced concentration or delayed excretion of tracer according to the method proposed by Schall and colleagues[37]

VI. Autoantibodies: presence in the serum of the following autoantibodies:

   1. Antibodies to Ro(SSA) or La(SSB) antigens, or both

---

symptoms, oral symptoms, and salivary gland dysfunction without the need for focal lymphocytic infiltrates or anti-Ro/La antibodies.[9] The AECG criteria modified this classification to include at least one objective finding, thus redefining the rules of the ESGCC.

When developing the 2002 AECG criteria, receiver operating characteristic (ROC) curves were constructed based on an analysis of 180 cases selected from a patient group provided by 16 centers from 10 European countries. The study group included 76 patients classified as having primary SS (pSS) by the judgment of the clinician, 41 patients with different CTDs without clinical evidence of secondary SS, and 63 patients with sicca complaints but no SS. The ROC analysis allowed for determination of the accuracy of different combinations of positive items to correctly classify patients (true positive patient cases) plus controls (true negative control cases) with respect to the total number of cases included in the study group.

The ROC analyses showed that using 4 of 6 positive elements to meet criteria, combinations that included only symptoms yielded greater sensitivities and lower specificities, whereas criteria sets that included only objective findings yielded lower sensitivities and higher specificities. The AECG agreed that combinations of subjective and objective parameters from the ROC curves should replace the previously proposed any 4 of 6 combination in classifying patients with pSS. The AECG subsequently decided that certain specifications must be added to the criteria sets in order to make the item definitions more precise and the tests more generally applicable (**Box 2**).

The AECG criteria set represents a combination of subjective assessments, objective salivary and ocular function tests, histopathology, and autoantibodies. Because some components of the

---

Box 2
Revised rules for classification for pSS

In patients without any potentially associated disease, pSS may be defined as follows:

a. The presence of any 4 of the 6 items indicates pSS, if either item IV (histopathology) or VI (serology) is positive

b. The presence of any 3 of the 4 objective criteria items (ie, items III, IV, V, and VI)

c. The classification tree procedure represents a valid alternative method for classification, although it should be more properly used in clinical-epidemiologic surveys

---

classification criteria could be met using multiple different tests (ie, item V, salivary gland involvement could be met by either unstimulated whole salivary flow rates, sialography changes, or scintigraphy), patients could meet classification of pSS having met 4 of the following 6 criteria:

1. Ocular symptoms
2. Oral symptoms
3. Ocular signs assessed by Schirmer I test or ocular dye scores
4. Histopathology
5. Salivary signs assessed by unstimulated whole salivary flow, positive parotid sialography, or positive salivary scintigraphy
6. Antibodies to Ro(SSA) or La(SSB) antigens, or both

The AECG also reached a consensus on a list of exclusion criteria (see **Box 2**) and criteria to classify cases of secondary SS (**Box 3**). The

---

Box 3
Revised rules for classification for secondary SS

In patients with a potentially associated disease (eg, another well-defined CTD), the presence of item I or item II plus any 2 from among items III, IV, and V may be considered to indicate secondary SS

Exclusion criteria:

  Past head and neck radiation treatment

  Hepatitis C infection

  AIDS

  Preexisting lymphoma

  Sarcoidosis

  Graft-versus-host disease

  Use of anticholinergic drugs (since a time <4-fold the half-life of the drug)

---

group used for comparison in classifying secondary SS comprised 72 patients clinically classified as having SS associated with another well-defined disease CTD, and 41 patients with CTDs but clinically classified as not having secondary SS.

CRITIQUE OF THE AECG CRITERIA

The low numbers of patients used for this criteria development and the lack of geographic variety were a few of the overall criticisms of the AECG criteria. In the following list are other reported weaknesses, some of which were considered by the Sjögren's International Collaborative Clinical Alliance (SICCA) group in developing new criteria specific to the measures used.[21]

(Items 1 and 2) Ocular/oral symptoms*:

- Scales for scoring subjective measures vary and are not unique
- Subjective tests lack specificity for SS and do not correlate with objective measures
- The use of subjective tests potentially creates a heterogeneous pool of patients with SS, making it difficult to diagnose, assess efficacy of treatment, and determine the prognosis of patients with SS

*One strength was that symptoms are the usual prompts that drive patients to seek out a diagnosis.

(3) Ocular signs assessed by Schirmer I test

- The test does not correlate with disease
- The test lacks specificity for SS

(4) Ocular signs assessed by ocular dye scores

- This is a time-consuming grading system that is difficult to apply in clinical practice

(5) Histopathology: none found
(6) Salivary signs assessed by salivary flow rates

- Types of saliva (whole vs individual gland) and collection techniques (spitting, drooling, suction devices, absorption, use of wafers, use of iodine starch) vary
- Other factors such as circadian variation, patient hydration, fasting state, medication, and possibly age and sex affect saliva production rates
- Measures lack specificity for SS

(7) Salivary signs assessed by sialography

- Technique is becoming obsolete
- Technique cannot distinguish between various causes of glandular inflammation

(8) Salivary signs assessed by scintigraphy

- Test scores correlate with flow rates but not FSs
- The test may not provide sufficient diagnostic specificity to offset monetary expenses
- The test lacks specificity for SS
- The test requires referral to a tertiary-care facility and placement of intravenous access for radiographic dye isotope placement

(9) Autoantibodies

- Found in only 60% of patients with SS
- Found in other CTDs
- The presence of these autoantibodies correlates with earlier onset of the disease, longer duration of SS, and is associated with extraglandular features (parotid gland enlargement, vasculitis, splenomegaly)[22]

ACR CRITERIA

SICCA was funded by the National Institutes of Health to develop new classification criteria for SS, citing "The need for new classification criteria is clear considering the current lack of standardization inherent to the use of multiple older criteria in the field, and the emergence of biological agents as potential treatments,"[21] and that "considering the potentially serious adverse effects and comorbidities of these agents, criteria used for enrollment into clinical trials will need to be clear, easy to apply, and have high specificity. They also must rely upon well-established objective tests that are clearly associated with the systemic/autoimmune, oral, and ocular characteristics of the disease, and include alternate tests only when they are diagnostically equivalent." The SICCA group also states that it would be desirable for new classification criteria for SS to be endorsed by professional rheumatology organizations across the world (such as the ACR or European League Against Rheumatism [EULAR]) to increase their credibility and maximize standardization when enrolling participants into clinical trials.

The SICCA group used consensus methodology derived from the nominal group technique.[23] This included defining the target population, identifying an initial list of criteria components and selection of preliminary classification criteria. Validation exercises were then performed.

These criteria were developed in 4 phases. An expert panel was convened in 2004 made up of members the relevant clinical specialties (7 rheumatologists, 6 ophthalmologists, and 7 experts in oral medicine) from a heterogeneous geographic area (9 members [45%] were from the United States; the rest were from 4 countries on 3 continents) to review evidence-based literature and to generate items. There was a consensus that panel members would use objective tests (eg, specific serum measures of autoimmunity, ocular staining reflecting lacrimal hypofunction, and LSG biopsy reflecting focal lymphocytic sialadenitis) that would likely be part of the new classification criteria. It was agreed that no diagnostic labels would be used for enrollment and that all participants would undergo the same set of standardized objective tests and questionnaires capturing various signs and symptoms. The final list of potential criteria items is available at http://sicca.ucsf.edu/.

Data analysis summaries were presented to the group by the epidemiologist. Cutoff values for tests were set, and possible surrogates were discussed. Frequency tables, binary regression, classification trees, and Venn diagrams were generated. Results from a statistical classification based on latent class analysis were presented to the panel of experts and represented a subset of participants (n = 1107). Classification criteria target individuals with signs and symptoms that may be suggestive of SS such as previous suspicion or diagnosis of SS, increased serum autoantibody levels; bilateral parotid enlargement, a recent increase in dental caries; or have diagnoses of RA or SLE. The rationale for these eligibility criteria was that only patients with such characteristics would be evaluated for SS or considered for enrollment in a clinical trial designed to evaluate a potential therapeutic agent for SS.

The final criteria were selected (**Box 4**) and criteria validation was made by comparison with a gold standard diagnosis derived from a statistical model fitted to data from a range of diagnostic tests rather than comparisons with patients diagnosed with the disease by clinical judgment. External validation was performed on approximately 300 participants not included in the original data set. Controls were selected among participants observed to be negative according to the AECG criteria (participants with RA, SLE, scleroderma, or other CTD were excluded from these analyses).

ACR CRITERIA CRITIQUE

Criticisms of the ACR criteria start with the method with which patients were identified, because no preliminary definition of the disease was provided. In addition, there are a few examples of classification criteria for rheumatic diseases derived by applying the methodology used to derive this criteria.[24] As more validation exercises are

---

Box 4
ACR classification criteria for SS[a]

The classification of SS, which applies to individuals with signs/symptoms that may be suggestive of SS, is met in patients who have at least 2 of the following 3 objective features:

1 Positive serum anti-SSA (Ro) or anti-SSB (La) or (positive RF and ANA $\geq$1:320)

2 Labial salivary gland biopsy showing focal lymphocytic sialadenitis with an FS of 1 focus/4 mm^2 or greater[b]

3 Keratoconjunctivitis sicca with ocular staining score of 3 or greater (assuming that individual is not using daily eye drops for glaucoma and has not had corneal surgery or cosmetic eyelid surgery in the last 5 years)[c]

Previous diagnosis of any of the following conditions excludes participation in SS studies or therapeutic trials because of overlapping clinical features or interference with criteria tests:

• History of head and neck radiation treatment

• Hepatitis C infection

• AIDS

• Sarcoidosis

• Amyloidosis

• Graft-versus-host disease

• IgG4-related disease

[a] Exclusion: participants with RA, SLE, scleroderma, or other CTD from the analyses, because there were only 87 (6%) such participants.
[b] Using histopathologic definitions and FS assessment methods previously described and OSS previously described.[30]
[c] Using ocular staining score as previously described.[27]

---

performed using the ACR criteria, more information will be brought forth to determine the performance of this methodology.

Usually, when developing new criteria sets, proposed criteria sets are compared with a gold standard. The practice of defining a gold standard is based on a series of cases (those with the disease) and controls (those without the disease) identified by expert clinicians. The investigators of the ACR criteria acknowledge that although this is the system that is generally used, it was not practical for them to apply this to their methodology "because diagnosis must rely on three clinical specialties." In this case, comparisons were made to alternative versions of the preliminary criteria, derived from a statistical model fitted to data rather than to patients with diagnosed pSS.

Another criticism of the ACR criteria was that patients with SS and another associated systemic autoimmune disorder (secondary SS) were excluded from the analyses. Nevertheless, the preliminary criteria were proposed as a valid tool to classify secondary SS even although it is established that patients with secondary SS tend to manifest different patterns of clinical presentation.[24]

Although in theory, the ACR criteria claim to be a simple criteria set because they include only 3 objective items, they may be more difficult for the general practitioner to apply. Research centers may have a readily available network of easily accessible rheumatologists, oral medicine specialists, and ophthalmologists, but this may not be feasible in the private practice setting. The Schirmer I test could be easily administered in the rheumatology or dental office setting. Under the new criteria, patients need to be referred to an ophthalmologist who is familiar with the scoring system, resulting in possible delay or inaccuracies in assessment.

Another concern regarding the criteria selected by the ACR was that patients with low ocular flow who have may not yet have progressed to surface abrasion as well as patients with low salivary flow without lymphocytic infiltrates (possibly because of error in sampling or errors in scoring inflammation, for example) or those patients with subclinical immunologic processes may be misclassified. It is possible that these patients are at an earlier stage of the disease or may have subclinical immunologic processes and may have a higher likelihood of response to treatments.[24] Daniels reports that within the SICCA population with keratoconjunctivitis sicca (KCS) only at baseline, a few people developed features of SS 2 years later.[25] In addition, it has been postulated that abnormal FS and presence of anti-SSA/SSB autoantibodies might not be independent variables, that there is some interdependency of the classification criteria, which increases the probability of not classifying cases of SS with a negative biopsy or autoantibodies.[26]

With regards to the ocular stain scoring (OSS) method used in the ACR criteria, a new method was developed by Whitcher and colleagues,[27] which is a modification of the Oxford scoring system developed by Bron and colleagues[28] for assessing KCS. This new method was tested on the same population with SICCA used for development of the ACR criteria. This new scoring system also gives equal weight of corneal (0–6) staining to conjunctiva staining (nasal 0–3; temporal 0–3). There was no explanation of how the OSS cutoff of 3 or higher was determined or why corneal staining could now account for half of the maximal score ($\leq$6), whereas in previous ocular scoring methods, corneal staining accounted for one-third of the total score. Although this scoring system was compared with tear breakup time and Schirmer I scores, it was not compared with Oxford scores[28] or van Bjisterveld scores.[29] It is therefore impossible to compare this scoring system with previously established systems and results. Also, exclusion criteria in the Witcher study did not mention those individuals who had punctual occlusion, those already on medications such as cyclosporine eye drops or other eye lubricants, or those taking parasympathomimetics. The scoring system proposed by Witcher used Venn diagrams to visualize the interrelationships between an abnormal OSS and the other 2 main phenotypic characteristics of SS (FS and serology), the investigators used an FS of greater than 1 rather than FS 1 or greater to classify patients.

With regards to the laboratory items selected by SICCA, criteria included a combination of alternative, less specific measures (ANA and RF) in place of more specific measures (SSA and SSB autoantibodies) derived by a consensus decision rather than the stated purposes for establishment of new classification criteria, and eliminated the Schirmer test from the objective eye criteria because of its lower specificity compared with ocular staining.[24]

In diagnosing SS, there are potentially many subclinical immunologic processes that precede clinical disease, potentially delaying diagnosis by several years or preventing patients from entry in clinical trials while at an early disease stage when they have a greater potential for response to biologics. If establishing classification criteria is intended to allow monitoring for changes

caused by a therapeutic intervention, many innovative tests or other such candidate markers for SS such as α-fodrin autoantibodies, M_3 receptor antibody, ultrasonography, magnetic resonance imaging (MRI), and MRI sialography may have been better candidates for consideration.[30] Following these markers or imaging may be more reflective of response to biologics in clinical trials than the ones selected.

COMPARISON OF AECG WITH ACR CRITERIA IN CLINICAL PRACTICE

In order to determine the usefulness of the ACR criteria in a clinical practice, we examined 100 consecutive patients who met the AECG at the Sjögren's Syndrome and Salivary Disorders Center, Carolinas Center for Oral Health, Carolinas Health Care System, Charlotte, NC. As shown in **Table 1**, the specific criteria used in the ACR classification criteria (ie, serology, ocular staining, and labial salivary gland biopsy) were documented based on the available data of 100 patients with pSS based on the AECG criteria. Of the 100 patients with pSS based on the AECG criteria, only 5 patients had sufficient data available to meet the ACR criteria (**Table 1**).

There are a numerous reasons that only 5 of 100 patients with pSS by the AECG criteria would also meet the ACR criteria with the data available in this particular clinical practice. First, this oral medicine practice receives many referrals from rheumatologists in the community to further evaluate for pSS, when patients have negative laboratory test results but still have symptoms and extraglandular manifestations suggestive of pSS. Only 24 of 100 patients had either a positive

Table 1
Number (%) of patients with pSS meeting or diagnosed by the A–E criteria who met specific ACR criteria and classified by the ACR criteria as SS

Sjögren Criteria	Positive	Negative	Completed but not Scored by Criteria	Not Completed or not Available
Meets A-E[a] criteria	100	0	—	—
Meets ACR criteria	5	95	—	—
Specific ACR criteria				
Serum				
Anti-SSA or anti-SSB positive	24	72	—	4
ANA $\geq$1:320 and +RF	3	86	—	11
OSS: lissamine green on the conjunctiva and fluorescein on the cornea	2	2	3	93
Labial salivary gland biopsy: focal lymphocytic sialadenitis/FS $\geq$1/4 mm^2	75	1	0	24

[a] A-E, American-European criteria.

anti-SSA or anti-SSB, therefore a minor salivary gland biopsy was completed in these patients with negative autoimmune serology. Approximately 60% of pSS have positive laboratory test results, therefore there is a referral bias with this present sample with only 24% having a positive laboratory test result. In addition, the 24 patients with positive laboratory test results did not have the minor salivary gland biopsy completed, because these patients met the AECG criteria without this additional invasive test. Theoretically, if the rate of positive laboratory test results was higher (eg, 60%) in this patient population, most of these patients would likely meet the AECG criteria and would not require a salivary gland biopsy to meet the classification criteria.

The lower rate of positive autoimmune serology is not the main reason for the lower rate of AECG positive patients with pSS also meeting the ACR criteria. The primary factor is the challenges of obtaining ocular staining scores, as proposed in the ACR criteria. Only 4 of 100 patients had staining scored in a manner consistent with the ACR criteria, whereas another 3 of 100 had staining but it was not scored in a way that could be used by the ACR criteria. The remaining 93 patients did not have ocular staining completed, or no eye examination was available for assessment. All 100 patients did have a Schirmer I test available, but this is not used in the ACR criteria.

DISCUSSION

The purpose of classification criteria is to separate patients with a disease both from patients without the disease and from normal individuals. Conceptually, classification criteria become, in practice, the same as diagnostic criteria. There are examples in the scientific literature in which some have attempted to determine if a certain classification criteria set is the best way to diagnose SS.[30] In a perfect world, if sensitivity and specificity were both 100%, they would be termed diagnostic criteria. However, classification criteria sets are not perfect, and a certain proportion of patients are always misclassified. Thus, criteria committees should be careful to emphasize that meeting (or not meeting) classification criteria does not equate to a diagnosis and that the physician, considering features of an individual patient beyond those represented in the criteria, is the only one who can establish a diagnosis for an individual patient.[1]

One potential source of confusion that the ACR criteria present is that because they are endorsed by the ACR, these classification criteria have the potential to be more frequently confused with diagnostic criteria, which has occurred with other autoimmune conditions. According to Tsuboi and colleagues,[31] the ACR revised criteria for the classification of SLE (1997) have been adopted for establishing diagnosis in daily clinical practice as well as for classification purposes in clinical studies. Tsuboi and colleagues also assert that the 2010 RA classification criteria (an ACR/EULAR collaborative initiative) is used not only in clinical studies of RA but also in daily clinical practice for the diagnosis of RA. Therefore, these diagnostic systems for SLE and RA could be regarded as the gold standard for both clinical studies and daily clinical practice.

If ACR classification criteria are adopted as diagnostic criteria, this may have a great impact on the reported prevalence of the disease. As Baldini and colleagues reported,[26] when criteria sets switch to the use of more objective measures, the overall prevalence of pSS estimated according to the preliminary European criteria varied from a minimum of 0.35 (95% confidence interval [CI], 0.17–0.65) to a maximum of 3.59 (95% CI, 2.43–5.08). Classified using the AECG criteria, the prevalence estimates decreased to 0.05 (95% CI, 0.048–0.052) to 0.6 (95% CI, 0.24–1.39).[32–35] The higher stringency allowed the AECG criteria to identify more homogeneous patients, but the higher specificity was extensively criticized. There have been no published prevalence estimates using the ACR criteria, but with the increased strictness of the ACR criteria, it will be interesting to see the overall prevalence estimates of SS with this newer classification criteria.

If the ACR criteria are used to estimate prevalence rates of SS and the prevalence is greatly reduced, this may have an impact on the willingness of drug companies to pursue SS as a new indication for existing drugs or the development of novel therapies.

Decreased prevalence rates may also have an impact on insurance coverage, both medical and dental, for patients.

In addition, the use of ocular staining alone in the ocular assessment may cause delays in classifying those with SS. With AECG criteria, ocular involvement could be assessed by the Schirmer I test without anesthesia. This procedure could be performed in the clinical setting of the rheumatologist or the oral medicine specialist. The ACR criteria would require patients to be referred to an ophthalmologist, specifically one with knowledge of the scoring system developed by the SICCA group. Because this scoring system is new, it will be an additional challenge to find ophthalmologists who are familiar with this scoring system for individuals or group practices not affiliated with a clinical trial consortium.

Classification criteria will continue to change as technology advances and knowledge of SS increases. This progress will make a more homogeneous patient population and it is hoped lead to earlier diagnosis and development of more effective therapeutics. However, it is possible that newly established criteria sets may not allow for direct comparison between new studies and previous ones.

REFERENCES

1. Fries JF, Hochberg MC, Medsger TA Jr, et al. Criteria for rheumatic disease. Different types and different functions. The American College of Rheumatology Diagnostic and Therapeutic Criteria Committee. Arthritis Rheum 1994;37(4):454–62.

2. Bloch KJ, Buchanan WW, Wohl MJ, et al. Sjoegren's syndrome. A clinical, pathologic, and serologic study of sixty-2 cases. Medicine 1965;44:187–231.

3. Daniels TE, Silverman S Jr, Michalski JP, et al. The oral component of Sjogren's syndrome. Oral Surg Oral Med Oral Pathol 1975;39(6):875–85.

4. Homma M, Tojo T, Akizuki M, et al. Criteria for Sjogren's syndrome in Japan. Scand J Rheumatol Suppl 1986;61:26–7.

5. Manthorpe R, Frost-Larsen K, Isager H, et al. Sjogren's syndrome. A review with emphasis on immunologic features. Allergy 1981;36(3):139–53.

6. Skopouli FN, Drosos AA, Papaioannou T, et al. Preliminary diagnostic criteria for Sjogren's syndrome. Scand J Rheumatol Suppl 1986;61:22–5.

7. Fox RI, Robinson CA, Curd JG, et al. Sjogren's syndrome. Proposed criteria for classification. Arthritis Rheum 1986;29(5):577–85.

8. Vitali C, Bombardieri S, Moutsopoulos HM, et al. Preliminary criteria for the classification of Sjogren's syndrome. Results of a prospective concerted action supported by the European Community. Arthritis Rheum 1993;36(3):340–7.

9. Vitali C, Bombardieri S, Jonsson R, et al. Classification criteria for Sjogren's syndrome: a revised version of the European criteria proposed by the American-European Consensus Group. Ann Rheum Dis 2002;61(6):554–8.

10. Shearn MA. Major problems in internal medicine. Sjogren's syndrome, vol. 2. Philadelphia: WB Saunders; 1971.

11. Ohfuji T. Sjogren's Disease Research Committee. Review on research reports: annual report of the Ministry of Health and Welfare. Japan: Japanese Ministry of Health; 1977.

12. Fujibayashi T. Revised diagnostic criteria for Sjogren's Syndrome. Rheumatology: Oxford; 2000.

13. Guellec D, Cornec D, Jousse-Joulin S, et al. Diagnostic value of labial minor salivary gland biopsy for Sjogren's syndrome: a systematic review. Autoimmun Rev 2013;12(3):416–20.

14. Takeda Y, Komori A. Focal lymphocytic infiltration in the human labial salivary glands: a postmortem study. J Oral Pathol 1986;15(2):83–6.

15. Stewart CM, Bhattacharyya I, Berg K, et al. Labial salivary gland biopsies in Sjogren's syndrome: still the gold standard? Oral Surg Oral Med Oral Pathol Oral Radiol Endod 2008;106(3):392–402.

16. Tavoni AG, Baldini C, Bencivelli W, et al. Minor salivary gland biopsy and Sjogren's syndrome: comparative analysis of biopsies among different Italian rheumatologic centers. Clin Exp Rheumatol 2012;30(6):929–33.

17. Harley JB, Alexander EL, Bias WB, et al. Anti-Ro (SS-A) and anti-La (SS-B) in patients with Sjogren's syndrome. Arthritis Rheum 1986;29(2):196–206.

18. Research in dry eye: report of the Research Subcommittee of the International Dry Eye Workshop (2007). Ocul Surf 2007;5(2):179–93.

19. Yavuz B, Bozdag Pehlivan S, Unlu N. An overview on dry eye treatment: approaches for cyclosporin a delivery. TheScientificWorldJournal 2012;2012:194848.

20. Murray Thomson W, Chalmers JM, John Spencer A, et al. A longitudinal study of medication exposure and xerostomia among older people. Gerodontology 2006;23(4):205–13.

21. Shiboski SC, Shiboski CH, Criswell L, et al. American College of Rheumatology classification criteria for Sjogren's syndrome: a data-driven, expert consensus approach in the Sjogren's International Collaborative Clinical Alliance cohort. Arthritis Care Res (Hoboken) 2012;64(4):475–87.

22. Tzioufas AG, Voulgarelis M. Update on Sjogren's syndrome autoimmune epithelitis: from classification to increased neoplasias. Best Pract Res Clin Rheumatol 2007;21(6):989–1010.

23. Fink A, Kosecoff J, Chassin M, et al. Consensus methods: characteristics and guidelines for use. Am J Public Health 1984;74(9):979–83.

24. Vitali C, Bootsma H, Bowman SJ, et al. Classification criteria for Sjogren's syndrome: the authors actually need to definitively resolve the long debate on the issue. Ann Rheum Dis 2013;72(4):476–8.

25. Daniels TE. Do the authors need new diagnostic criteria for Sjogren's syndrome? Presse Med 2012;41(9 Pt 2):e441–9.

26. Baldini C, Talarico R, Tzioufas AG, et al. Classification criteria for Sjogren's syndrome: a critical review. J Autoimmun 2012;39(1–2):9–14.

27. Whitcher JP, Shiboski CH, Shiboski SC, et al. A simplified quantitative method for assessing keratoconjunctivitis sicca from the Sjogren's Syndrome International Registry. Am J Ophthalmol 2010;149(3):405–15.

28. Bron AJ, Evans VE, Smith JA. Grading of corneal and conjunctival staining in the context of other dry eye tests. Cornea 2003;22(7):640–50.

29. van Bijsterveld OP. Diagnostic tests in the Sicca syndrome. Arch Ophthalmol 1969;82(1):10–4.

30. Aframian DJ, Konttinen YT, Carrozzo M, et al. Urban legends series: Sjogren's syndrome. Oral Dis 2013; 19(1):46–58.

31. Tsuboi H, Hagiwara S, Asashima H, et al. Validation of different sets of criteria for the diagnosis of Sjogren's syndrome in Japanese patients. Mod Rheumatol 2013;23(2):219–25.

32. Binard A, Devauchelle-Pensec V, Fautrel B, et al. Epidemiology of Sjogren's syndrome: where are the authors now? Clin Exp Rheumatol 2007;25(1):1–4.

33. Goransson LG, Haldorsen K, Brun JG, et al. The point prevalence of clinically relevant primary Sjogren's syndrome in 2 Norwegian counties. Scand J Rheumatol 2011;40(3):221–4.

34. Haugen AJ, Peen E, Hulten B, et al. Estimation of the prevalence of primary Sjogren's syndrome in 2 age-different community-based populations using 2 sets of classification criteria: the Hordaland Health Study. Scand J Rheumatol 2008;37(1):30–4.

35. Mavragani CP, Moutsopoulos HM. The geoepidemiology of Sjogren's syndrome. Autoimmun Rev 2010; 9(5):A305–10.

36. Rubin P, Holt JF. Secretory sialography in diseases of the major salivary glands. American Journal of Roentgenology, Radium Therapy, and Nuclear Medicine 1957;77(4):575–98.

37. Schall GL, Anderson LG, Wolf RO, et al. Xerostomia in Sjogren's syndrome. Evaluation by sequential salivary scintigraphy. JAMA 1971;216(13):2109–16.

Salivary Gland Biopsy for Sjögren's Syndrome

Konstantina Delli, DDS, MSc, Dr med dent,
Arjan Vissink, DDS, MD, PhD, Fred K.L. Spijkervet, DMD, PhD*

KEYWORDS

• Salivary gland • Biopsy • Labial gland • Parotid gland • Sjögren's syndrome

KEY POINTS

- Lymphocytic sialadenitis in labial salivary glands is a widely accepted criterion for histologic confirmation of Sjögren's syndrome (SS).
- Sensitivity and specificity of parotid and labial biopsies for diagnosing SS are comparable.
- Parotid gland incision biopsy can overcome most of the disadvantages of labial gland excision biopsy.
- In contrast to labial salivary glands, lymphoepithelial lesions and early stage lymphomas can often be observed in parotid gland tissue of patients with SS.
- Parotid tissue can be harvested easily; repeated biopsies from the same parotid gland are possible; histopathologic results can be compared with other diagnostic results derived from the same gland.
- Parotid biopsies, in contrast to labial salivary gland biopsy, allow the clinician to prospectively monitor disease progression and to assess the effects of the intervention treatment at a glandular level.

INTRODUCTION

Salivary gland biopsy is a technique broadly applied for the diagnosis of Sjögren's syndrome (SS), lymphoma accompanying SS, sarcoidosis, amyloidosis, and other connective tissue disorders. SS has characteristic microscopic findings involving lymphocytic infiltration surrounding the excretory ducts in combination with the destruction of acinar tissue (**Fig. 1**). In affected parotid glands, epimyoepithelial islands in a background of lymphoid stroma can be additionally seen, and lymphoepithelial lesions (LELs) are a common phenomenon (**Fig. 2**).

Biopsy of the labial salivary glands is considered one of the 4 objective American-European Consensus Group's (AECG) classification criteria and one of the 3 objective American College of Rheumatology's (ACR) classification criteria for SS (**Table 1**). Although the parotid biopsy has been shown to be an alternative for labial salivary gland biopsy when applying the AECG's classification criteria, it has yet to be validated in regard to the ACR's classification criteria.[1]

This article focuses on the main techniques used for taking labial and parotid salivary gland biopsies in the diagnostic workup of SS with respect to their advantages, their postoperative complications, and their usefulness for diagnostic procedures, monitoring disease progression, and treatment evaluation.

LABIAL SALIVARY GLAND BIOPSY

Minor salivary glands are widely distributed in the labial, buccal, and palatal mucosa of the oral cavity.[2] Because pathognomonic changes are seen in minor salivary glands, the minor salivary gland biopsy is largely used for assisting the diagnosis of SS. Labial salivary glands, in particular, are easily accessible, lie above the muscle layer, and are separated from the oral mucous membrane by a

Department of Oral and Maxillofacial Surgery, University Medical Center Groningen, University of Groningen, Groningen, the Netherlands
* Corresponding author. Department of Oral and Maxillofacial Surgery, University Medical Center Groningen, PO Box 30.001, 9700 RB Groningen, The Netherlands.
E-mail address: f.k.l.spijkervet@umcg.nl

Oral Maxillofacial Surg Clin N Am 26 (2014) 23–33
http://dx.doi.org/10.1016/j.coms.2013.09.005
1042-3699/14/$ – see front matter © 2014 Elsevier Inc. All rights reserved.

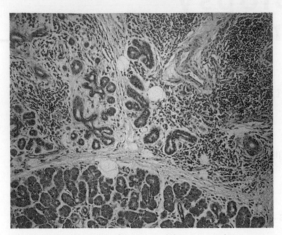

Fig. 1. Lymphocytic infiltration (*) surrounding excretory ducts and destruction of acini (Hematoxylin and Eosin stain (H&E)).

thin layer of fibrous connective tissue. Although the chance of excessive bleeding is minimal, because the arterial supply to the lip lies deep,[3] there is a risk of sensible nerve injury because the branches of the mental nerve in the lower lip are closely associated to the minor salivary glands (**Fig. 3**).[4]

Labial salivary gland biopsies in the diagnosis of SS were introduced by Chisholm and Mason[5] in 1968 and involved oral preparation of patients with local anesthetic infiltration followed by excising an ellipse of oral mucous membrane down to the muscle layer.[5] The wound was closed with 4-0 silk sutures, which were removed after 4 to 5 days. Ideally, 6 to 8 minor glands must be harvested and sent for histopathologic examination.

Several technicians have revised this technique (**Table 2**). Greenspan and colleagues[6] described a 1.5- to 2.0-cm linear incision of mucosa, parallel to the vermillion border and lateral to the midline.

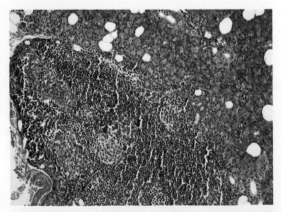

Fig. 2. Lymphoepithelial lesions (*) form as the result of atrophy of the columnar ductal epithelium and proliferation of basal epithelial cells, associated with intraepithelial infiltration. (*Courtesy of* Dr EA Haacke)

Marx and colleagues[7] modified Greenspan's technique with a mucosal excision of 3.0 × 0.75 cm. Delgado and Mosqueda[8] preferred a longitudinal incision of 1 cm in the labial mucosa in front of the mandibular cuspids. Guevara-Gutierrez and coworkers[9] proposed the punch biopsy technique performed with a 4-mm punch just penetrating the epithelium of the lower lip. Mahlsted and colleagues[10] recommended a 1.0- to 1.5-cm wedge-shaped excision of mucosa between the midline and commissure. Gorson and Ropper[11] reported a 1-cm vertical incision just behind the wet line through the mucosa and submucosa. An oblique incision, starting 1.5 cm from the midline and proceeding latero-inferiorly, avoiding the glandular-free zone in the center of the lower lip was advocated by Berquin and colleagues.[12] Caporali and colleagues[13] reported a small incision of 2 to 3 mm on the inner surface of the lower lip. In view of the lack of sufficient evidence to support the superiority of one technique over the others, especially in respect to short- and long-term morbidity, the shape and the size of the incision can be considered a matter of preference. The incision shape has included elliptical, horizontal, vertical, and wedge shapes; the incision length has varied from a few millimeters to 2 cm. The authors of the present article, based on their clinical experience, suggest a horizontal incision of approximately 2 cm, which is in agreement with the technique proposed by Greenspan and colleagues[6] whereby the surgeon uses loupe operation glasses (magnification × 2.5) to precisely excise the salivary glands without disturbing the direct underlying sensible nerves (**Fig. 4**).

The first grading system for salivary gland biopsies was used by Chisholm and Mason[5] in an attempt to standardize the examined area and record the degree of histopathologic change. At present, according to the revised AECG's classification criteria and the ACR's classification criteria for SS, a labial salivary gland biopsy is considered positive if minor salivary glands (obtained through normal-appearing mucosa) demonstrate focal lymphocytic sialadenitis, evaluated by an expert histopathologist, with a focus score of 1 or more (defined as several lymphocytic foci, containing more than 50 lymphocytes per 4 mm^2 of glandular tissue) (see **Table 1**).

Complications

The most commonly reported complications of labial gland biopsy are the following[1,6–8,10,12–17]:

1. Localized sensory alteration (frequently described with the terms *anesthesia*, *reduced or*

Table 1
Histologic criteria for diagnosing SS on salivary gland biopsies

Type of Biopsy	Positivity
Labial gland	If minor salivary glands (obtained through normal-appearing mucosa) demonstrate focal lymphocytic sialadenitis, evaluated by an expert histopathologist, with a focus score 1 or more, defined as several lymphocytic foci (which are adjacent to normal appearing mucous acini and contain more than 50 lymphocytes) per 4 mm^2 of glandular tissue
Parotid gland	If one of the 2 following criteria is fulfilled: 1. A focus score of 1 or more, defined as the number of lymphocytic foci (which are adjacent to normal-appearing acini and contain >50 lymphocytes) per 4 mm^2 of glandular parotid tissue (including fat tissue), regardless of the presence of benign LELs 2. Small lymphocytic infiltrates, not fulfilling the criterion of a focus score of more than 1, in combination with the presence of benign LELs
Sublingual	Not determined

Abbreviation: LELs, lymphoepithelial lesions.
Data from Refs.[1,18,19]

partial loss of sensation, transitory numbness, and *hypoesthesia*); may last for a few months or can be permanent
2. External hematoma
3. Local swelling
4. Formation of granulomas
5. Internal scarring and cheloid formation
6. Falling sutures
7. Local pain

Suitability for Diagnostic and Treatment Evaluation Purposes

A widely accepted criterion for histologic confirmation of SS is focal lymphocytic sialadenitis in labial salivary glands.[18,19] Labial biopsies are mainly well suited for the diagnostic workup but

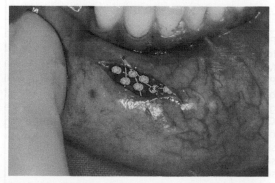

Fig. 3. The branch of the mental nerve (*) that supplies the mucous membrane of the lower lip usually divides into 2 sub-branches (a horizontal and a vertical), which have an ascending course toward the vermillion border and are in close relation to the labial salivary glands (**).

not for treatment and disease activity evaluation[20]; although very rare, B-cell mucosa-associated lymphoid tissue (MALT) lymphomas can be found in labial biopsies of patients with SS.[21,22]

PAROTID GLAND BIOPSY

The parotid gland is the largest salivary gland and is positioned on the lateral aspect of the face overlying the posterior surface of the mandible and anteroinferior to the auricle.[23] Traditionally, the gland is divided into a superficial and deep lobe based on the course of the facial nerve as it passes through. When the facial nerve enters the parotid gland, it forms a characteristic branching pattern that resembles a goosefoot and is known as the *pes anserinus*, giving 2 main divisions of the facial nerve (**Fig. 5**). Surgically, the facial nerve can be located in approximately 2 to 4 mm deep to the inferior end of the tympanomastoid suture line and 1 cm deep and slightly anteroinferior to the tragal pointer.

Kraaijenhagen[24] initially described the parotid gland biopsy technique: the area is anesthetized with local infiltration anesthesia after the standard preparation. With a No. 15 blade, a small 1- to 2-cm incision is made just below the earlobe near the posterior angle of the mandible. The skin is incised, and the parotid capsule is exposed by blunt dissection. The capsule of the gland is carefully opened, and a small amount of superficial parotid tissue is removed. The procedure is completed with a 2- to 3-layered closure. The capsule must be cautiously closed to avoid future leakage or the development of sialocele (**Fig. 6**).

The technique was slightly modified by the present authors with an incision below and slightly

Table 2
Comparison of techniques

	Technique	Advantages	Complications
Labial gland			
Chisholm & Mason,[5] 1968	Ellipse of oral mucous membrane down to the muscle layer; harvest of 6 to 8 glands; wound closure with 04-gauge silk sutures, which must be removed after 4 to 5 days	1. Widely distributed glands 2. Easily accessible glands 3. Minimal chance of bleeding	1. Temporary or permanent alteration in sensation in the area of the incision 2. External hematoma 3. Local swelling 4. Granulomas formation 5. Internal scarring and cheloid formation 6. Suture failing 7. Local pain
Greenspan et al,[6] 1974	1.5- to 2.0-cm linear incision of mucosa, parallel to the vermillion border and lateral to the midline		
Marx et al,[7] 1988	Mucosal incision of 3.0 × 0.75 cm		
Delgado & Moscueda,[8] 1989	Longitudinal incision of 1 cm in the labial mucosa in front of the mandibular cuspids		
Guevara-Gutierrez et al,[9] 2001	Punch biopsy		
Mahlsted et al,[10] 2002	1.0- to 1.5-cm wedge-shaped incision between the midline and commissure		
Gorson & Ropper,[11] 2003	1-cm vertical incision just behind the wet line through the mucosa and submucosa		
Berquin et al,[12] 2006	Oblique incision, starting 1.5 cm from the midline and proceeding latero-inferiorly, avoiding the glandular-free zone in the center of the lower lip		
Caporali et al,[13] 2007	Small incision of 2 to 3 mm on the inner surface of the lower lip		
Parotid gland			
Kraaijenhagen,[24] 1975 Marx et al,[7] 1988 McGuirt et al,[43] 2002 Baurmash et al,[44] 2005 Pijpe et al,[1] 2007	1- to 2-cm incision just below and behind the earlobe near the posterior angle of the mandible; the skin is incised and the parotid capsule is exposed by blunt dissection; capsule of the gland is opened and adequate amount of superficial parotid tissue is removed; the procedure is completed with a 2- to 3-layered closure	1. Presence of LELs 2. Identification of MALT 3. Possibility of repeated biopsy from the same gland 4. Comparison with other diagnostic results derived from the same gland (eg, secretory function, sialographic appearance)	1. Temporary alteration in sensation in the area of the incision 2. Facial nerve damage 3. Sialoceles 4. Salivary fistulae 5. Risk of harvesting only fat tissue 6. Demanding surgical expertise

(continued on next page)

Table 2
(continued)

	Technique	Advantages	Complications
Sublingual salivary gland			
Pennec et al,[27] 1990 Adam et al,[28] 1992 Berquin et al,[12] 2006	Incision between the first premolar and the lateral cutting tooth	1. Collection of sufficient amount of tissue	1. Uncomfortable scars 2. Bleeding 3. Swelling in the floor of the mouth 4. Risk of ligaturing Wharton duct 5. Not established histopathologic criteria

Data from Refs.[5–13,24,27,28,43]

behind the earlobe (**Fig. 7**). The capsule of the parotid gland and subcutaneous tissue is closed with 4-0 Vicryl (Johnson & Johnson Inc, Belgium) sutures, whereas the skin is closed with 5-0 Ethilon sutures (Johnson & Johnson Inc, Belgium). In this way, the aesthetic results are excellent and future scar is invisible to the eye from an anterior/lateral point of view.

Pijpe and coworkers[1] established a new set of validated histopathologic criteria for diagnosing SS according to the AECG's classification criteria based on the biopsy of the parotid gland (see **Table 1**). A parotid biopsy was considered positive if one of the 2 following criteria was fulfilled:

1. A focus score of 1 or more (defined as the number of lymphocytic foci, which are adjacent to normal-appearing acini and contain >50 lymphocytes) per 4 mm^2 of glandular parotid tissue (including fat tissue), regardless of the presence of benign LELs
2. Small lymphocytic infiltrates, not fulfilling the criterion of a focus score of 1 or more, in combination with the presence of benign LELs

Complications

Despite the potential risk of facial nerve damage and the development of sialoceles and salivary fistulae, a temporary change in sensation in the skin area of the incision is the only well-documented complication described to date.[1,7]

Suitability for Diagnostic and Treatment Evaluation Purposes

Parotid biopsies allow the clinician to monitor the disease progression and to assess the effect of

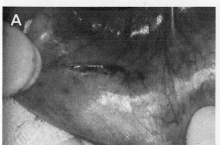
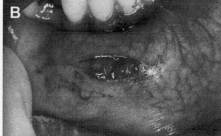
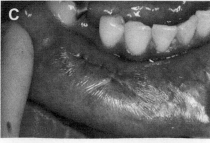

Fig. 4. Harvesting labial salivary glands. (*A*) Horizontal incision of approximately 1.5 cm. (*B*) Harvest of 6 to 8 minor salivary glands. (*C*) Closure of the wound with 5-0 Vicryl (Johnson & Johnson Inc, Belgium) rapide (resorbable) inverted, buried notch sutures.

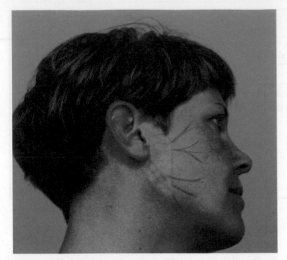

Fig. 5. The facial nerve enters the parotid gland forming a characteristic branching pattern that resembles a goosefoot and is known as the *pes anserinus*, giving 2 main divisions of the facial nerve. The parotid gland is divided into a superficial and deep lobe based on the course of the facial nerve as it passes through. In the area of the incisional biopsy of the parotid gland, the distance between the gland surface and the facial nerve is approximately 1.5 cm.

an intervention treatment in SS. This is feasible because parotid tissue can be harvested easily, repeated biopsies from the same parotid gland are possible, and the histopathologic results can

be compared with other diagnostic results derived from the same gland (eg, secretory function, sialographic appearance, and ultrasound).[25] Additionally, by performing parotid biopsies as a routine diagnostic procedure for SS, LELs and lymphomas located in the parotid gland can identified.[7,26]

SUBLINGUAL SALIVARY GLAND BIOPSY

The sublingual salivary gland is the smallest of the major salivary glands. It lies in the floor of the mouth on both sides of the tongue and is covered only by oral mucosa. There are a few reports about taking a biopsy of the sublingual salivary gland for the diagnosis of SS.[12,27,28] The technique is performed with a 1-cm linear mucosal incision in the floor of the mouth, 1 cm anterolaterally from the Wharton duct to 1 cm anteroposteriorly.[12,27,28]

Complications

The postoperative complications of sublingual salivary gland biopsy are the following[12,27]:

1. Ligaturing the Wharton duct, resulting from the placement of sutures
2. Bleeding
3. Swelling in the floor of the mouth

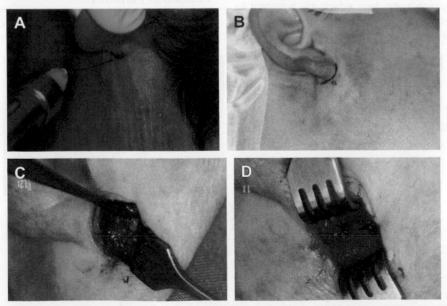

Fig. 6. Incisional biopsy of the parotid gland. (*A*) The area is anesthetized with local infiltration anesthesia. (*B*) With a No. 15 blade, a small 1- to 2-cm incision is made just below and behind the earlobe near the posterior angle of the mandible. (*C*) The skin is incised, and the parotid capsule is exposed by blunt dissection. The capsule of the gland is carefully opened, and a small amount of superficial parotid tissue is removed. (*D*) The procedure is completed with a 2- to 3-layered closure with 4-0 absorbable sutures (polyglycolic acid), and the skin layer is closed with 5-0 nylon sutures.

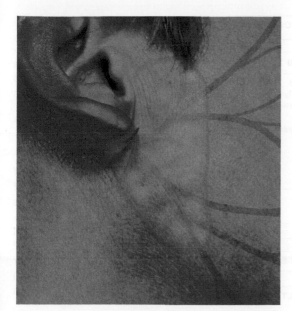

Fig. 7. The technique of the biopsy of the parotid gland was slightly modified by the present authors with an incision below and slightly behind the earlobe (*blue line*).

COMPARISON OF TECHNIQUES

Although focal lymphocytic sialadenitis in the labial salivary gland is a widely accepted criterion for histologic confirmation of SS, biopsies of the labial salivary glands may have several disadvantages (**Table 2**). The sensitivity and specificity of labial salivary gland biopsies vary in the literature. Data from different studies are often difficult to compare because different sets of criteria for diagnosing SS have been used and the outcome of the labial biopsy is a strong determinant for the final diagnosis. In a normal population, the labial biopsy resulted in a 6% to 9% false-positive diagnoses; 18% to 40% of the patients with a clinical diagnosis of SS have a negative labial biopsy, resulting in a sensitivity of 60% to 82% and a specificity of 91% to 94% (**Table 3**).[14,29–33] According to the ACR's classification criteria, the labial biopsy has a sensitivity of 89.8% (95% confidence interval [CI] 87.2–92.0) but a lower specificity of 74.3% (95% CI 71.0–77.5).[19] Moreover, it may be difficult to harvest a sufficient number of labial salivary glands in atrophic submucosa of patients with longstanding SS.[30] In addition, permanent sensory loss of the mucosa of the lower lip, occurring in 1% to 10% of the patients, is a known complication of a labial biopsy[7,14,15] Pijpe and coworkers[1] report sensory loss in 6% of patients after labial biopsy, whereas no permanent sensory loss was observed after a parotid biopsy.

Table 3
Sensitivity and specificity of biopsy techniques

Technique	Sensitivity (%)	Specificity (%)
Labial gland biopsy	60–82	91–94
Parotid gland biopsy	78	86
Sublingual gland biopsy	66	52

Data from Pijpe J, Kalk WW, van der Wal JE, et al. Parotid gland biopsy compared with labial biopsy in the diagnosis of patients with primary Sjögren's syndrome. Rheumatology 2007;46:335–41; and Pennec YL, Leroy JP, Jouquan J, et al. Comparison of labial and sublingual salivary gland biopsies in the diagnosis of Sjögren's syndrome. Ann Rheum Dis 1990;49:37–9.

Incisional biopsy of the parotid gland can overcome most of the disadvantages of the labial biopsy (see **Table 2**). When evaluating the parotid and the labial biopsy, sensitivity and specificity are comparable (see **Table 3**), estimated to be 78% and 86%, respectively.[1] Parotid gland tissue can be harvested easily; repeated biopsies from the same parotid gland are possible (an important asset in studies assessing the efficacy of a treatment in patients with SS or monitoring disease progression); the histopathologic results can be compared with other diagnostic results derived from the same gland (secretory function, sialographic appearance, ultrasound). In contrast to labial salivary glands, LELs are often observed in the parotid gland tissue of patients with SS. These LELs, a characteristic histologic feature of the major salivary glands in SS,[33] develop as a result of hyperplasia of ductal basal cells within a lymphocytic infiltrate. In addition, well-formed lymphoid follicles or germinal centers, often adjacent to ductal epithelium, can be found in the major salivary glands.[34] Because both LELs and reactive lymphoid follicles also indicate malignant lymphoma, benign LELs must be discriminated from premalignant lesions using strict criteria.[35,36]

Four percent to 7% of patients with SS develop malignant B cell lymphoma,[37,38] 48% to 75% of which are of the MALT type. These B-cell lymphomas are most frequently located in the parotid gland.[39–41] The assessment of patients with SS who may have developed a MALT lymphoma is not always easy, but an incisional biopsy of the parotid gland can be safely performed under local anesthesia[4] and can help toward this diagnosis. Pollard and coworkers[26] have established an algorithm for the management of MALT-type lymphoma of parotid gland and associated SS (MALT-SS), showing the importance of a parotid gland biopsy for controlling the disease (**Fig. 8**).

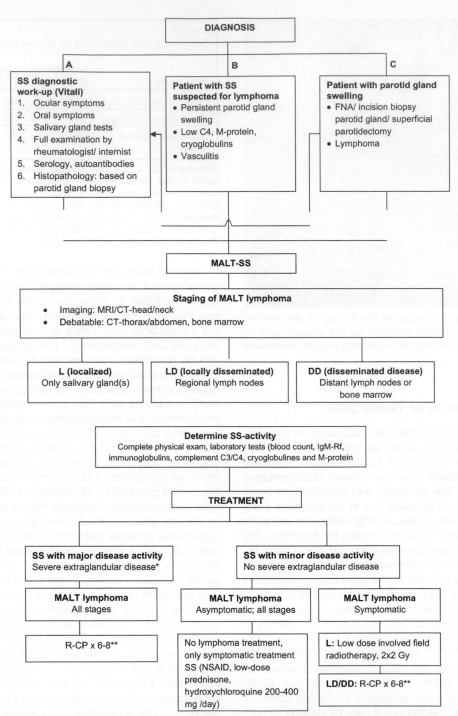

Fig. 8. Management of MALT-type lymphoma of parotid gland associated with SS (MALT-SS). *Severe extra-glandular disease: polyarthritis/myositis, glomerulonephritis, nervous system involvement, cryoglobulinemic vasculitis, other severe organ involvement, serologic abnormalities: cryoglobulinemia, C4 less than 0.10 g/L. **Six intravenous infusions of 375 mg/m² of rituximab and 6 to 8 cycles of cyclophosphamide, given every 3 weeks. FNA, fine-needle aspiration; IgM, immunoglobulin M; NSAID, nonsteroidal antiinflammatory drugs; R-CP, rituximab with cyclophosphamide and prednisone. (*Adapted from* Pollard RP, Pijpe J, Bootsma H, et al. Treatment of mucosa-associated lymphoid tissue lymphoma in Sjogren's syndrome: a retrospective clinical study. J Rheumatol 2011;38:2205; with permission.)

Additionally, in pediatric patients with clinical suspicion of SS and a negative minor salivary gland biopsy result, a parotid gland biopsy could be safe and effective in order to establish histopathologic evidence for the diagnosis of SS.[42]

Finally, it is noteworthy that the pain following labial and parotid biopsies is comparable in severity and disappears within 1 month.[1]

Notwithstanding these aforementioned advantages, biopsies of the parotid gland have not become commonplace because of the concern for damage to the facial nerve and the development of sialoceles and salivary fistulae (see **Table 2**). In addition, parotid gland biopsies are not part of the established criteria for diagnosing SS and demand higher surgical expertise. They are validated for the AECG's classification criteria but not yet for the ACR's classification criteria.

A comparison of sublingual gland biopsy with labial gland biopsy has shown that the sensitivity of sublingual gland biopsy is better than that of the labial gland biopsy, whereas the specificity of the latter is better than that of the former (see **Table 3**).[27] As far as the postoperative complications are concerned, researchers claim that sublingual gland biopsy is a relatively safe procedure (see **Table 2**). Because placing a suture might increase the risk of ligaturing the Wharton duct and lead to swelling of the floor of the mouth, no suture[28] or careful placement of 1 to 2 sutures could be an alternative.[29] Damage to the mental nerve is obviously not feasible because of the operation site, whereas damage to the lingual nerve related to this biopsy technique has never been reported in the literature. An advanced risk of bleeding is encountered in cases when a more posterior incision is made, which, however, resolves spontaneously.[12] To date, specialized histopathologic criteria have not been established for the diagnosis of SS after a sublingual gland biopsy, and researchers merely used the criteria for labial gland biopsies.[12,27,29]

SUMMARY

Early diagnosis and treatment are of high importance for preventing the complications associated with SS. Unfortunately, so far there is not a single test capable of confirming the diagnosis of SS. A positive salivary gland biopsy provides strong evidence, which, in correlation with additional diagnostic tests, can establish the classification of SS. Parotid gland biopsy is a relatively simple technique, has the potential to overcome most of the disadvantages of the labial biopsy, and can additionally aid in monitoring disease progression and the effect of an intervention treatment in SS.

REFERENCES

1. Pijpe J, Kalk WW, van der Wal JE, et al. Parotid gland biopsy compared with labial biopsy in the diagnosis of patients with primary Sjögren's syndrome. Rheumatology 2007;46:335–41.
2. Geerling G, Raus P. Minor salivary gland transplantation. Dev Ophthalmol 2008;41:243–54.
3. Meskin LH, Bernard B, Warwick WJ. Biopsy of the labial mucous salivary glands in cystic fibrosis. JAMA 1964;188:82–3.
4. Alsaad K, Lee TC, McCartan B. An anatomical study of the cutaneous branches of the mental nerve. Int J Oral Maxillofac Surg 2003;32:325–33.
5. Chisholm DM, Mason DK. Labial salivary gland biopsy in Sjögren's disease. J Clin Pathol 1968;21:656–60.
6. Greenspan JS, Daniels TE, Talal N, et al. The histopathology of Sjögren's syndrome in labial salivary gland biopsies. Oral Surg Oral Med Oral Pathol 1974;37:217–29.
7. Marx RE, Hartman KS, Rethman KV. A prospective study comparing incisional labial to incisional parotid biopsies in the detection and confirmation of sarcoidosis, Sjögren's disease, sialosis and lymphoma. J Rheumatol 1988;15:621–9.
8. Delgado WA, Mosqueda A. A highly sensitive method for diagnosis of secondary amyloidosis by labial salivary gland biopsy. J Oral Pathol Med 1989;18:310–4.
9. Guevara-Gutierrez E, Tlacuilo-Parra A, Minjares-Padilla LM. Minor salivary gland punch biopsy for evaluation of Sjögren's syndrome. J Clin Rheumatol 2001;7:401–2.
10. Mahlsted K, Ussmüller J, Donath K. Value of minor salivary gland biopsy in diagnosing Sjögren's syndrome. J Otolaryngol 2002;31:299–303.
11. Gorson KC, Ropper AH. Positive salivary gland biopsy, Sjögren syndrome, and neuropathy: clinical implications. Muscle Nerve 2003;28:553–60.
12. Berquin K, Mahy P, Weynand B, et al. Accessory or sublingual salivary gland biopsy to assess systemic disease: a comparative retrospective study. Eur Arch Otorhinolaryngol 2006;263:233–6.
13. Caporali R, Bonacci E, Epis O, et al. Comment on: parotid gland biopsy compared with labial biopsy in the diagnosis of patients with primary Sjögren's syndrome [author reply]. Rheumatology 2007;46:1625.
14. Daniels TE. Labial salivary gland biopsy in Sjögren's syndrome. Assessment as a diagnostic criterion in 362 suspected cases. Arthritis Rheum 1984;27:147–56.
15. Richards A, Mutlu S, Scully C, et al. Complications associated with labial salivary gland biopsy in the investigation of connective tissue disorders. Ann Rheum Dis 1992;51:996–7.

16. Friedman H, Kilmar V, Galletta VP, et al. Lip biopsy in connective tissue diseases. A review and study of seventy cases. Oral Surg Oral Med Oral Pathol 1979;47:256–62.

17. Teppo H, Revonta M. A follow-up study of minimally invasive lip biopsy in the diagnosis of Sjögren's syndrome. Clin Rheumatol 2007;26:1099–103.

18. Vitali C, Bombardieri S, Jonsson R, et al, European Study Group on Classification Criteria for Sjögren's Syndrome. Classification criteria for Sjögren's syndrome: a revised version of the European criteria proposed by the American-European Consensus Group. Ann Rheum Dis 2002;61:554–8.

19. Shiboski SC, Shiboski CH, Criswell L, et al, Sjögren's International Collaborative Clinical Alliance (SICCA) Research Groups. American College of Rheumatology classification criteria for Sjögren's syndrome: a data-driven, expert consensus approach in the Sjögren's International Collaborative Clinical Alliance cohort. Arthritis Care Res (Hoboken) 2012; 64:475–87.

20. Vissink A, Bootsma H, Kroese FG, et al. How to assess treatment efficacy in Sjögren's syndrome? Curr Opin Rheumatol 2012;24:281–9.

21. Van Mello NM, Pillemer SR, Tak PP, et al. B cell MALT lymphoma diagnosed by labial minor salivary gland biopsy in patients screened for Sjögren's syndrome. Ann Rheum Dis 2005;64:471–3.

22. Theander E, Vasaitis L, Baecklund E, et al. Lymphoid organisation in labial salivary gland biopsies is a possible predictor for the development of malignant lymphoma in primary Sjögren's syndrome. Ann Rheum Dis 2011;70:1363–8.

23. Witt RL. Salivary gland anatomy. In: Salivary gland diseases. Surgical and medical management. New York: Thieme Medical Publishers; 2005. p. 1–7.

24. Kraaijenhagen HA. Letter: technique for parotid biopsy. J Oral Surg 1975;33:328.

25. Pijpe J, Meijer JM, Bootsma H, et al. Clinical and histologic evidence of salivary gland restoration supports the efficacy of rituximab treatment in Sjögren's syndrome. Arthritis Rheum 2009;60: 3251–6.

26. Pollard RP, Pijpe J, Bootsma H, et al. Treatment of mucosa-associated lymphoid tissue lymphoma in Sjögren's syndrome: a retrospective clinical study. J Rheumatol 2011;38:2198–208.

27. Pennec YL, Leroy JP, Jouquan J, et al. Comparison of labial and sublingual salivary gland biopsies in the diagnosis of Sjögren's syndrome. Ann Rheum Dis 1990;49:37–9.

28. Adam P, Haroun A, Billet J, et al. Biopsy of the salivary glands. The importance and technic of biopsy of the sublingual gland on its anterio-lateral side. Rev Stomatol Chir Maxillofac 1992;93:337–40.

29. Lindahl G, Hedfors E. Focal lymphocytic infiltrates of salivary glands are not confined to Sjögren's syndrome. Scand J Rheumatol Suppl 1986;61: 52–5.

30. Vitali C, Tavoni A, Simi U, et al. Parotid sialography and minor salivary gland biopsy in the diagnosis of Sjögren's syndrome. A comparative study of 84 patients. J Rheumatol 1988;15:262–7.

31. De Wilde PC, Kater L, Baak JP, et al. A new and highly sensitive immunohistologic diagnostic criterion for Sjögren's syndrome. Arthritis Rheum 1989; 32:1214–20.

32. Vitali C, Moutsopoulos HM, Bombardieri S. The European Community Study Group on diagnostic criteria for Sjögren's syndrome. Sensitivity and specificity of tests for ocular and oral involvement in Sjögren's syndrome. Ann Rheum Dis 1994;53:637–47.

33. Ihrler S, Zietz C, Sendelhofert A, et al. Lymphoepithelial duct lesions in Sjögren-type sialadenitis. Virchows Arch 1999;434:315–23.

34. Jordan RC, Speight PM. Lymphoma in Sjögren's syndrome. From histopathology to molecular pathology. Oral Surg Oral Med Oral Pathol Oral Radiol Endod 1996;81:308–20.

35. Quintana PG, Kapadia SB, Bahler DW, et al. Salivary gland lymphoid infiltrates associated with lymphoepithelial lesions: a clinicopathologic, immunophenotypic, and genotypic study. Hum Pathol 1997;28: 850–61.

36. De Vita S, De Marchi G, Sacco S, et al. Preliminary classification of nonmalignant B cell proliferation in Sjögren's syndrome: perspectives on pathobiology and treatment based on an integrated clinico-pathologic and molecular study approach. Blood Cells Mol Dis 2001;27:757–66.

37. Sutcliffe N, Inanc M, Speight P, et al. Predictors of lymphoma development in primary Sjögren's syndrome. Semin Arthritis Rheum 1998;28:80–7.

38. Theander E, Henriksson G, Ljungberg O, et al. Lymphoma and other malignancies in primary Sjögren's syndrome: a cohort study on cancer incidence and lymphoma predictors. Ann Rheum Dis 2006;65: 796–803.

39. Kassan SS, Thomas TL, Moutsopoulos HM, et al. Increased risk of lymphoma in sicca syndrome. Ann Intern Med 1978;89:888–92.

40. Tzioufas AG, Boumba DS, Skopouli FN, et al. Mixed monoclonal cryoglobulinemia and monoclonal rheumatoid factor cross-reactive idiotypes as predictive factors for the development of lymphoma in primary Sjögren's syndrome. Arthritis Rheum 1996;39:767–72.

41. Voulgarelis M, Dafni UG, Isenberg DA, et al. Malignant lymphoma in primary Sjögren's syndrome: a multicenter, retrospective, clinical study by the European Concerted Action on Sjögren's syndrome. Arthritis Rheum 1999;42:1765–72.

42. Radfar L, Kleiner DE, Fox PC, et al. Prevalence and clinical significance of lymphocytic foci in minor

salivary glands of healthy volunteers. Arthritis Rheum 2002;47:520–4.

43. McGuirt WF Jr, Whang C, Moreland W. The role of parotid biopsy in the diagnosis of pediatric Sjögren syndrome. Arch Otolaryngol Head Neck Surg 2002;128:1279–81.

44. Baurmash H. Parotid biopsy technique. J Oral Maxillofac Surg 2005;63:1556–7.

Salivary Gland Dysfunction and Xerostomia in Sjögren's Syndrome

Siri Beier Jensen, DDS, PhD[a],*, Arjan Vissink, DMD, MD, PhD[b]

KEYWORDS

- Sjögren's syndrome • Salivary gland dysfunction • Hyposalivation • Sialometry • Xerostomia
- Subjective assessment

KEY POINTS

- Unstimulated whole saliva sialometry is a major criterion for evaluation of salivary gland dysfunction in Sjögren's syndrome according to the American-European Consensus Group classification criteria.
- Stimulated whole saliva sialometry and gland specific sialometry are of importance for diagnosing patients with SS. Unstimulated and stimulated sialometry are essential in identifying patients who may benefit from intervention therapy.
- Xerostomia should be assessed regularly by validated tools to evaluate impact on oral health-related quality of life and monitor alleviation/treatment efficacy or disease progression.

INTRODUCTION

It is generally accepted that the secretions of the salivary glands are of paramount importance for the maintenance of oral health. A reduced salivary flow induces symptoms that include the subjective feeling of dry mouth (xerostomia), difficulty with the swallowing of food, and an increased susceptibility to dental caries and opportunistic infections. These symptoms reflect the impact of reduced salivary flow on the maintenance of the health of the oral tissues, because salivary dysfunction negatively affects several main functions of saliva, such as (1) protecting the mineralized tissues against wear and demineralization, (2) wetting the oral mucosa, thereby forestalling oral desiccation and infection, and (3) promoting speech and the digestion of food. In this article, salivary gland dysfunction and xerostomia in Sjögren's syndrome (SS) is discussed, with a focus on the pathophysiology of salivary dysfunction in SS, the clinical presentation of dry mouth in SS, how to assess salivary gland hypofunction and xerostomia in SS, and the impact of salivary gland dysfunction on quality of life in patients with SS.

SALIVARY GLAND PHYSIOLOGY
What is Saliva?

The mixed fluid in the mouth is called whole saliva or oral fluid. Whole saliva is for the greater part composed of secretions from 3 pairs of major salivary glands (parotid, submandibular [SM], and sublingual [SL]) and from numerous minor glands (labial, buccal, lingual, palatal, retromolar). Each type of gland secretes a fluid with a characteristic protein composition.[1] In addition, whole saliva contains gingival crevicular fluid, microorganisms, food debris, and shed mucosal cells. Saliva is a hypotonic fluid relative to plasma, and it is composed of more than 99% water and less than 1% of dry matter, such as proteins and salts. The normal

a Section of Oral Medicine, Clinical Oral Physiology, Oral Pathology and Anatomy, Department of Odontology, Faculty of Health and Medical Sciences, University of Copenhagen, Nørre Allé 20, 2200 Copenhagen N, Denmark; b Department of Oral and Maxillofacial Surgery, University of Groningen and University Hospital Groningen, P.O. Box 30.001, 9700 RB Groningen, The Netherlands
* Corresponding author.
E-mail address: sirib@sund.ku.dk

Oral Maxillofacial Surg Clin N Am 26 (2014) 35–53
http://dx.doi.org/10.1016/j.coms.2013.09.003
1042-3699/14/$ – see front matter © 2014 Elsevier Inc. All rights reserved.

daily production of whole saliva ranges between 0.5 and 1.5 L.

At night and in resting state during daytime, the SM and SL glands are the main contributors to whole saliva (**Table 1**). Together with the numerous minor salivary glands, they secrete most of the salivary mucins.[2] The large salivary mucins are responsible for the viscoelastic properties of mucous saliva. These large glycoproteins are the backbone of the lubricating layers that cover all oral surfaces, acting as diffusion barriers impeding the entry of noxious agents, including acids, microorganisms, and viruses. This mucous layer helps in reducing the friction between antagonistic tooth surfaces. The low-molecular-weight mucins have broad-spectrum bacteria-binding properties and play an important role in the oral clearance of bacteria, yeasts, and viruses. Without mucins, the oral mucosa and the dental surfaces become highly vulnerable to infection, inflammation, and mechanical wear.[3]

Saliva Secretion: The Two-Step Model

Basically, saliva is formed in 2 steps. The secretory end pieces (acini) produce primary saliva, which is isotonic, having an ionic composition similar to that of plasma (**Fig. 1**). The primary fluid is then modified in the ductal system by selective reabsorption of sodium and chloride, and by a certain secretion of potassium and bicarbonate, although the duct is impermeable to water. Thus the secretion rate and thereby the volume of final saliva are determined directly by the formation rate of primary saliva by the acinar cells.

The ionic composition of saliva is strongly dependent on the secretion rate. When the salivary secretion rate is low (eg, at rest), the mouth fluid is rich in potassium and chloride and low in sodium and bicarbonate. On stimulation of the flow rate, sodium, chloride, and bicarbonate concentrations increase, and potassium decreases (**Fig. 2**). This situation can be explained by the ion exchange mechanism during saliva transport in the ductal system, in particular during its transport in the striated ducts. Similar to the fluid secreted by most exocrine organs (eg, sweat and lacrimal glands), saliva formation involves 2 stages. The primary fluid secreted by salivary acinar cells resembles plasma in ionic composition, which is rich in sodium, chloride, and bicarbonate (see **Fig. 1**). As this primary secretion passes through the ductal system, sodium, chloride, and bicarbonate are reabsorbed, whereas potassium is excreted, resulting in a fluid hypotonic to plasma, although rich in potassium. When saliva secretion rate is increased, as a result of the combination of a maximum reabsorption capacity in the duct epithelium and the shorter passage time in the duct, the stimulated saliva secretion is less hypotonic than the resting saliva. This situation results in apparently increased sodium, chloride, and bicarbonate concentrations and decreased potassium concentration.

Stimulation of salivary secretions thus influences both the quantity of saliva and its ionic and protein composition. In addition, large differences exist between individuals, both in the volume and the protein composition of saliva. Altogether this situation makes it difficult, in particular for whole saliva, to define normal reference values for salivary parameters with which to compare patient data.

Salivary Secretion and Composition in SS

When discussing whole saliva, one should be aware that saliva enters the mouth at several locations, but the different glandular secretions are not well mixed. For example, the contribution of parotid saliva to (un)stimulated whole saliva varies from site to site, ranging from being the major contributor to whole saliva collected buccally from the maxillary molars to being almost noncontributing to whole saliva collected in the incisor region. This site-specific variation in composition of whole saliva seems to account for the site specificity of smooth surface caries and supragingival

Table 1
Relative (%) contribution of different gland types to whole saliva under various conditions

Salivary Gland	Sleep	Unstimulated Whole Saliva	Stimulated (Mechanical) Whole Saliva	Stimulated (Acid) Whole Saliva
Parotid	0	21	58	45
SM	72	70	33	45
SL	14	2	2	2
Minor glands	14	7	7	8

Data from Refs.[39–41]

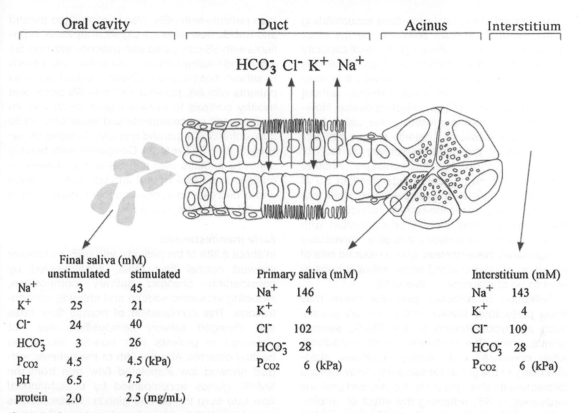

| Oral cavity | Duct | Acinus | Interstitium |

HCO_3^- Cl^- K^+ Na^+

Final saliva (mM)		Primary saliva (mM)		Interstitium (mM)	
	unstimulated	stimulated			
Na^+	3	45	Na^+ 146	Na^+	143
K^+	25	21	K^+ 4	K^+	4
Cl^-	24	40	Cl^- 102	Cl^-	109
HCO_3^-	3	26	HCO_3^- 28	HCO_3^-	28
P_{CO2}	4.5	4.5 (kPa)	P_{CO2} 6 (kPa)	P_{CO2}	6 (kPa)
pH	6.5	7.5			
protein	2.0	2.5 (mg/mL)			

Fig. 1. Ionic and protein composition of tissue fluid, acinar secretion, and oral fluid. (*From* Bardow A, Pedersen AM, Nauntofte B. Saliva. In: Miles TS, Nauntofte B, Svensson P, editors. Clinical oral physiology. 1st edition. Copenhagen (Denmark): Quintessence; 2004. p. 25; with permission.)

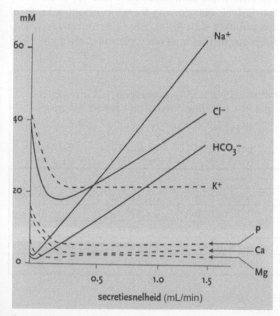

Fig. 2. Composition of saliva changes when salivary flow rate increases.

calculus deposition. The wide variation in local contribution of the various salivary glands to whole saliva is also obvious when assessing mucosal wetness, because the thickness of the salivary layer on the oral mucosa is thinner in the labial and anterior hard palatal region than on the buccal mucosa and anterior tongue.[4] This finding may explain the site-specific differences in oral dryness as reported by some patients.

In many studies, whole saliva is used, which has potential value in estimating which treatment might be effective in a particular patient with SS or for the use of saliva as a diagnostic tool in point-of-care diagnostics, because constituents from nonsaliva sources to whole saliva might be an asset in distinguishing patients with SS from patients with a salivary gland dysfunction mimicking SS. For understanding what is really happening regarding the salivary component of SS, analysis of glandular secretions, directly reflecting what is ongoing in a particular type of salivary gland, is preferred. Thus, in the assessment of the secretory capacity of a patient, a first glance measurement of the total secretions accumulating in the mouth (oral fluid) seems to be the most appropriate method, reflecting the overall capacity of all salivary glands. Collection of whole saliva is the method most often used, because it is easy to perform, taking only a few minutes, without the need for a specialized collecting device. However, for analytical purposes, whole saliva is of limited value, because it detects neither dysfunction of any of the separate salivary glands nor gland specific sialochemical changes. Another argument against its use in understanding SS at a glandular level is that whole saliva does not necessarily represent the sum of individual gland secretions but may include contamination with sputum, serum, food debris, and other nonsalivary components. Nevertheless, only a reduced rate of secretion of unstimulated whole saliva is considered to be of diagnostic value in SS.

Collection of selective glandular saliva may show preferential involvement of salivary glands, such as hyposalivation of the SM/SL salivary glands, which often is observed in SS. In addition, when compared with healthy individuals, sialochemistry of the glandular saliva may show several characteristic changes in electrolytes and proteins (enzymes) in SS, reflecting the effect of autoimmune attack on the secretory cells in individual salivary glands. However, in clinical practice, SS needs to be differentiated from other salivary gland diseases and conditions mimicking SS. When compared with healthy controls, salivary flow rate of patients with primary SS (pSS), patients with secondary SS (sSS), and patients with sicca complaints mimicking SS (non-SS sicca) is significantly lower (**Table 2**). Furthermore, patients with sSS have on average higher parotid flow rates

than patients with pSS. Also unstimulated parotid and SM/SL flow rates are significantly lower in patients with SS compared with patients with non-SS sicca and healthy controls. Moreover, with regard to salivary composition, differences exist between patients with SS, patients with non-SS sicca, and healthy controls to include higher mean sodium and chloride concentrations and lower phosphate concentrations in parotid and SM/SL saliva of patients with SS (**Table 3**). Compared with healthy controls, patients with non-SS sicca showed increases in potassium and amylase concentration and a decrease in sodium concentration, both in parotid and SM/SL saliva.

Early manifestations

In about a fifth of the patients with pSS, sialometry showed normal flow rates, accompanied by considerably changed salivary composition, including increased sodium and chloride concentrations. This combination of normal flow rates and changed salivary composition was not observed in patients with non-SS sicca and healthy controls. About a fifth of the patients with pSS showed low stimulated flow rate from the SM/SL glands accompanied by a (sub)normal flow rate from the parotid glands. These profiles are characteristic of early salivary manifestation of SS, because both occurred almost exclusively in the patients with SS and are related to short duration (<1 year) of oral symptoms.[5]

Late manifestations

Extremely low stimulated flow rate for exclusively the SM/SL glands was found in about a tenth of the patients with SS, whereas extremely low flow rates for all major salivary glands were found in a

Table 2
Salivary flow rate of SS-positive patients (groups A and B: pSS and sSS, respectively), SS-negative patients (patients suspected of having SS at referral, but not fulfilling the criteria for SS diagnosis, group C), and healthy controls (group D)

	Group A (n = 33)	Group B (n = 25)	Group C (n = 42)	Group D (n = 36)
Unstimulated				
Parotid flow rate (mL/min/gland)	0.02 (0.04)[a]	0.02 (0.04)[a]	0.04 (0.06)	0.05 (0.06)
SM/SL flow rate (mL/min/gland)	0.05 (0.09)[a,b]	0.02 (0.03)[a,b]	0.12 (0.13)	0.12 (0.12)
Stimulated				
Parotid flow rate (mL/min/gland)	0.12 (0.13)[a]	0.24 (0.25)[a]	0.19 (0.15)[a]	0.52 (0.42)
SM/SL flow rate (mL/min/gland)	0.24 (0.28)[a,b]	0.26 (0.35)[a]	0.42 (0.28)	0.46 (0.24)

Values are mean (standard deviation).
[a] Significant difference between patients and healthy controls. Statistical test used: analysis of variance.
[b] Significant difference between SS-positive and SS-negative patients.
Adapted from Kalk WW, Vissink A, Spijkervet FK, et al. Sialometry and sialochemistry: diagnostic tools for Sjögren's syndrome. Ann Rheum Dis 2001;60:1110–6; with permission.

Table 3
Composition of stimulated glandular saliva from SS-positive patients (groups A and B: pSS and sSS, respectively), SS-negative patients (patients suspected of having SS at referral, but not fulfilling the criteria for SS diagnosis, group C), and healthy controls (group D)

	Parotid Glands (Mean of Two Sides)				SM/SL Glands			
	Group A (n = 33)	Group B (n = 25)	Group C (n = 42)	Group D (n = 36)	Group A (n = 33)	Group B (n = 25)	Group C (n = 42)	Group D (n = 36)
Sodium (mmol/L)	26 (23)[a,b]	23 (22)[a]	4 (4)[b]	14 (12)	20 (15)[a,b]	16 (11)[a,b]	6 (6)[b]	11 (6)
Potassium (mmol/L)	23 (6)	23 (9)	30 (21)[b]	24 (6)	21 (21)	18 (7)	20 (6)[b]	17 (6)
Chloride (mmol/L)	30 (14)[b]	37 (28)[a,b]	18 (6)	16 (12)	27 (15)[b]	34 (35)[a,b]	16 (5)	16 (6)
Calcium (mmol/L)	1.3 (1.0)	1.0 (0.2)	1.3 (0.8)	0.8 (0.6)	1.9 (0.9)	1.9 (0.5)	2.2 (1.6)	1.7 (0.6)
Phosphate (mmol/L)	4.5 (2.4)	4.2 (1.6)	5.8 (2.9)	ND	2.3 (1.2)[a]	2.5 (1.2)[a]	3.9 (1.7)	ND
Urea (mmol/L)	5.6 (2.0)	4.9 (2.4)	6.1 (2.5)	3.8 (1.2)	2.9 (1.8)	3.8 (2.3)	4.0 (1.9)	2.5 (0.6)
Total protein (g/L)	1.2 (0.5)[b]	1.6 (1.3)[b]	1.2 (0.6)[b]	0.6 (0.6)	0.6 (0.3)	0.8 (0.5)	0.7 (0.4)	0.8 (0.6)
Total protein (g/min)	0.1 (0.1)	0.3 (0.5)	0.2 (0.2)	0.3 (0.3)	0.2 (0.2)	0.3 (0.6)	0.3 (0.3)	0.4 (0.3)
Amylase (10^3 U/L)	519 (344)	618 (474)	842 (486)[b]	590 (510)	117 (97)	162 (293)	138 (121)	ND
Amylase (10^3 U/min)	59 (65)	180 (295)	152 (142)	307 (264)	45 (60)	27 (60)	58 (70)	ND

Data are expressed as mean (standard deviation) and are based on the number of patients with available information.
Abbreviation: ND, not determined.
[a] Significant difference between SS-positive and SS-negative patients.
[b] Significant difference between patients and healthy controls. Statistical test used: analysis of variance (multicomparison according to Scheffé).
Adapted from Kalk WW, Vissink A, Spijkervet FK, et al. Sialometry and sialochemistry: diagnostic tools for Sjögren's syndrome. Ann Rheum Dis 2001;60:1110–6; with permission.

quarter (pSS, 30%; sSS, 16%). Extremely low flow rates for all salivary glands were rarely observed in patients with non-SS sicca and not in healthy controls. These profiles were related significantly to long duration (>2 years) of oral symptoms.[5]

What can saliva tell about the progression of SS?
As mentioned earlier, sialometry and sialochemistry can be used as a diagnostic tool either by collecting whole saliva (the combined secretions of all salivary glands) or by collecting glandular saliva (gland specific saliva). Although unstimulated whole saliva is a major criterion for evaluation of salivary gland dysfunction in SS, when SS develops, not all major salivary glands may yet manifest dysfunction, rendering whole saliva less valuable as a diagnostic tool or as a parameter for evaluating progression of the disease or therapeutic intervention than glandular saliva.[6,7] In contrast to whole saliva, analysis of gland specific

saliva can reveal sequential involvement of particular glands, reflecting the ongoing autoimmune process in individual major salivary glands. By using glandular saliva, patients with SS may frequently be diagnosed at an earlier stage, and progression or effects of therapeutic intervention can be measured in a noninvasive way (**Fig. 3**). This finding is also in agreement with studies showing progressive destruction of salivary gland tissue in patients with longer disease duration.[7]

Determination of glandular flow rates is not only important in the diagnostic workup of SS but it is, possibly, a parameter for assessing the potential for intervention.[7] Furthermore, patients with early SS have the highest sodium concentrations, which are related to more severe disease manifestations.[8] This finding argues for early diagnosis and immediate treatment of patients with early-onset pSS, who often have residual salivary gland function and high degrees of fatigue. An intervention study with B-cell depletion in patients with SS

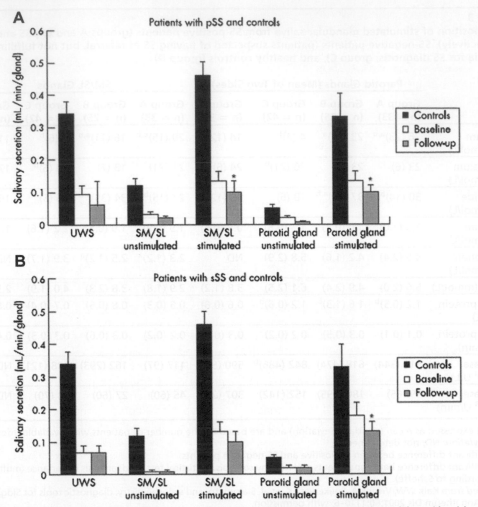

Fig. 3. Mean (standard error of the mean) salivary flow rates of patients with pSS (*A*), sSS (*B*), and healthy controls at baseline and 3.6 ± 2.3 (mean ± standard deviation) years follow-up. UWS, unstimulated whole saliva. *$P<.05$ versus baseline, by Wilcoxon signed rank. (*From* Pijpe J, Kalk WW, Bootsma H, et al. Progression of salivary gland dysfunction in patients with Sjögren's syndrome. Ann Rheum Dis 2007;66:107–12; with permission.)

showed that only patients with sufficient residual gland function (ie, patients with early SS) responded well to treatment.[9] It seems that some residual salivary gland tissue is necessary for either recovery or regeneration of secretory gland tissue after intervention therapy. Therefore, gland specific sialometry is not only of paramount importance for diagnosing patients with early-onset SS but also crucial in identifying patients who may benefit highly from intervention therapy.

PATHOPHYSIOLOGY OF SALIVARY GLAND DYSFUNCTION AND XEROSTOMIA IN SS

SS is considered to be an autoimmune disorder. Arguments for the autoimmune pathogenesis are the presence of characteristic autoantibodies, the strong female preponderance, the association

with HLA-DR3/B8, the association with other systemic and organ-specific autoantibodies, and the histopathologic findings in the affected glands.

As for the etiopathogenesis of SS, no definite answers are as yet available, comparable with other autoimmune diseases. Various findings have suggested that viruses may be involved, in particular the Epstein-Barr virus, the Coxsackie virus, and retroviruses such as human T-lymphotropic virus 1. However, these findings have not been convincingly confirmed. Some virus infections, in particular hepatitis C virus and human immunodeficiency virus infection, can produce symptoms and pathologic findings similar to that in SS. However, the presence of these latter infections is an exclusion criterion for SS. Besides these exogenous factors, various endogenous factors may be involved, in particular, hormonal factors, apparent from the strong female preponderance and genetic factors. The extended haplotype HLA-DR3/B8/DQ-2, in combination with the C4A null gene, is present in around 50% of patients with SS compared with 20% to 25% of controls. Thus, both exogenous and endogenous factors could be involved in the cause of SS, but no single factor is apparent.[10]

The pathologic findings in the affected glands may give a clue to the pathogenetic pathways involved in the development of the characteristic inflammatory SS lesion. T cells (80%), particularly CD4-positive T cells, predominate in the infiltrates, and recent data, as in other autoimmune diseases, suggest that CD4-positive Th-17 cells secreting interleukin 17 are major effector cells in the glands.[11] In addition, clusters of B cells, constituting 10% to 20% of the infiltrate, as well as plasma cells are present. Like all cells that belong to the mucosal immune system, the salivary glands of healthy individuals contain mostly IgA-producing B cells and plasma cells. However, the B cells and plasma cells in the glands of patients with SS produce predominantly IgG, with a local production of autoantibodies. Depletion of B lymphocytes using a CD20-specific monoclonal antibody (rituximab) resulted in improvement of salivary function in patients with recent-onset pSS, as well as restoration, at least in part, of the architecture of the ductal system in the parotid gland.[9,12] This finding suggests that B cells play a major pathogenic role in disease development. The precise mechanisms leading to glandular destruction in SS have not been fully elucidated.

The pathogenetic pathways operative in the salivary glands could also be operative in other organs affected in SS, such as the lungs and kidneys, in which CD4-positive interstitial infiltrates may occur. Besides, small-vessel vasculitis can be present in SS. This feature is clinically manifest as purpura in the skin, mononeuritis multiplex, and glomerulonephritis. Here, deposition of immune complexes consisting of mixed cryoglobulins is considered a major pathogenic factor.

As mentioned earlier, SS is a lymphoproliferative disease, in which B cells play a dominant role. Severe hypergammaglobulinemia and the presence of various autoantibodies are serologic hallmarks of the disease. Monoclonal components are frequently present, both as circulating monoclonal antibodies in plasma and in the glandular tissues, as shown by molecular analysis of B cells. Increased production of B-cell activation factor by, among others, T cells may underlie B-cell proliferation.[13] This situation may lead to the development of B-cell lymphoma within the salivary glands as well as in other locations.

CLINICAL PRESENTATION OF DRY MOUTH

Dry mouth is rarely an isolated symptom. Usually, it is accompanied by other oral, as well as systemic, complaints. The oral symptoms primarily accrue from chronic salivary gland hypofunction, which induces, over time, a decrease in the amount and composition of the oral fluids that bathe and protect the oral tissues and contribute to the alimentary and masticatory functions of saliva. Patients may complain of dryness that is present throughout their oral cavity or of dryness that it is localized to select areas of the mouth (eg, the lips, cheeks, tongue, palate, floor of the mouth, and throat). They may also complain of difficulty with chewing, swallowing, and speaking. The general complaint as well as the severity of oral dryness is not proportionally related to a decrease in the flow rate of saliva.[14] In about a quarter of the patients complaining of moderate to severe oral dryness, the mouth might even appear moist on clinical inspection. However, salivary flow may sometimes be directly associated with other oral complaints. For example, the complaints of oral dryness while eating, the need to sip liquids to swallow food, or difficulties in swallowing have all been highly correlated with measurable decreases in the rate of flow of stimulated whole saliva. It is the stimulated saliva that is directly related to alimentation, mastication, and deglutition.

Dry mouth is also frequently associated with generalized desiccation. Patients should, therefore, be systematically queried about the presence of dryness in other body sites, especially the eyes, but also the throat, the nose, the skin, and the vaginal area. Most patients carry bottles of water or other fluids with them at all times to aid speaking and swallowing and for their overall oral comfort. The mucosa may be sensitive to spicy or coarse foods. This sensitivity limits the patient's enjoyment of meals and may compromise their nutrition. Other complaints that might be relevant in diagnosing the symptoms underlying the patients' perception of oral dryness are dry, tickling coughs, recurrent swelling of the major salivary glands, chronic fatigue, and painful joints.

Most patients with advanced salivary gland hypofunction have obvious signs of mucosal dryness. The lips often appear cracked, peeling, and atrophic. The buccal mucosa may appear pale and corrugated; the tongue may be smooth and reddened, with loss of some of the dorsal papillae, or may have, as commonly seen in patients with SS, a fissured appearance (**Fig. 4**). There is often a marked increase in erosion and dental caries, particularly recurrent lesions and

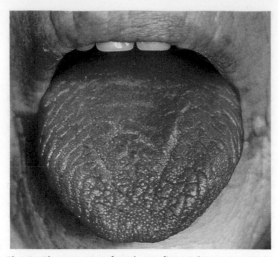

Fig. 4. The tongue often has a fissured appearance in patients with SS.

decay on root surfaces and even cusp tip involvement (**Fig. 5**). The decay may be progressive, even in the presence of vigilant oral hygiene. With diminished salivary output, there is a tendency for greater accumulations of food debris in the interproximal regions, especially where recession has occurred.

Candidiasis is frequent. It may appear as red, erythematous patches on the oral mucosa (eg, beneath dentures) or it may appear as white, curd-like mucocutaneous lesions on any surface (thrush). Fungal lesions of the corners of the mouth (angular cheilitis) are more likely to occur in patients with dry mouth who wear dentures and have a posterior bite collapse.

The patient should be examined for facial asymmetry. Enlargement of the salivary glands is frequently seen. The major salivary glands should be palpated to detect masses (eg, mucosal-associated lymphoid tissue lymphomas, non-Hodgkin lymphomas).

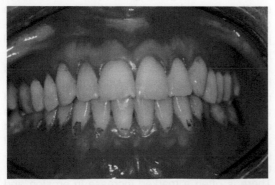

Fig. 5. Carious destruction of teeth in patients with SS often starts at the cervical region of teeth.

ASSESSMENT OF SALIVARY GLAND HYPOFUNCTION AND XEROSTOMIA

Along with assessing salivary gland hypofunction and xerostomia to establish an SS diagnosis, assessing the level of salivary gland hypofunction is also an asset in the treatment of xerostomia and salivary gland hypofunction. This treatment should be based on answers to the following:

- To determine the cause of the dry mouth. If the cause can be determined, eliminate it. This may abate the problem. It also may diminish the symptoms that are consequentially associated with it.
- To determine, if the cause cannot be assessed or if treating the cause only partially relieves the oral dryness, whether it is possible to stimulate the flow of saliva. This strategy, per se, may readily diminish the oral desiccation.
- To determine, if the saliva cannot be adequately stimulated, whether one can combat the arid feeling by coating the surfaces of the oral mucosa.
- To determine what else can be done to preserve and protect the teeth and the oral soft tissues and provide relief to the patient.

The most important issue that can be learned from this approach is that subjective and objective evaluation of both the pattern of complaints and the level of residual flow is of utmost important in both diagnosing the underlying cause of salivary gland dysfunction and selecting the most effective treatment option to prevent or reduce the causes and consequences of the dysfunction.

How to Measure Salivary Gland Hypofunction?

The single, most constant feature of saliva is its variability. Its volume, its composition, and its viscosity fluctuate throughout the day. Its normal values vary widely among individuals. The unstimulated secretion is significantly influenced by the time of day and year (circadian rhythms), by previous stimulation, by the position of the body, and by exposure to light and temperature. These are important, controllable variables, which should be standardized for each patient when conducting sialometric tests. Uncontrollable variables that affect flow include the gender, age, and weight of the patient, the size of the salivary glands, the patient's physical and mental health, and their intake of medications.[15]

As discussed earlier, the criteria used for the collection of saliva should be standardized for every patient. Regardless of the test used, the most critical of these factors is the time of day that the saliva sample is obtained and the length of the collection procedure. It is best if the sample can be obtained from a patient after an overnight fast. This is a readily duplicable event. The next best and more comfortable time for both the patients and clinician to routinely collect saliva is in the morning, between 8 and 11 AM. The patient must refrain from eating, drinking, smoking, or oral hygiene procedures for at least 90 minutes before the test session. Whatever the time set, whether after a fast or in the morning or even in the afternoon, the test should be performed as constantly as possible for each patient every time. Furthermore, the more time is taken to collect a sample of saliva, the more reliable it is. The minimum time is 5 minutes, but recent studies advocate 10 minutes for diagnostic and research purposes.[16] In the European Union–US criteria for SS, a collection time of 15 minutes for unstimulated whole saliva is required; the cutoff value is less than 1.5 mL/15 min (**Fig. 6**).[6]

Collection of Resting Whole Saliva

The flow rate of resting whole saliva can be performed by 4 techniques: the draining method, the spitting method, the suction method, and the swab technique. All of them provide roughly similar results; the swab technique is the least reliable. In the draining method, saliva is allowed to passively drain from the mouth into a collecting vessel (see **Fig. 6**). The spitting technique is similar to the draining method, but the accumulated saliva is periodically expectorated into a tube. The suction method involves the use of the standard, plastic, dental saliva ejector, and the swab method is conducted by placing preweighed cotton rolls or gauze sponges into the mouth, leaving them for a fixed period, and then reweighing them after the test. The swab method is an effective way to estimate the degree of salivation in patients with severe xerostomia. However, again, regardless of the method used, the conditions of the test should be the same for each patient each time that saliva is collected. The objective should be patient standardization.[15]

Collection of Stimulated Whole Saliva

Whole saliva is generally stimulated by either mastication or taste (see **Fig. 6**). One method uses chewing to stimulate saliva; the other, citric acid. Both methods are reliable. Flow rates using citric acid are generally greater than those induced by wax. When applying the masticatory method, the patient is either given a piece of paraffin wax (weight ~1–2 g; melting point 42°C–44°C), a piece of gum base, or a piece of Parafilm (Parafilm® M, Bemis Company, Inc, Neenah, Wisconsin, USA) to chew for 5 minutes. The accumulated saliva is

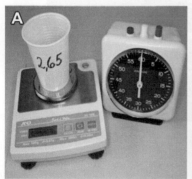 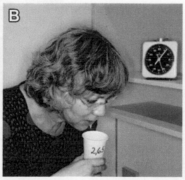 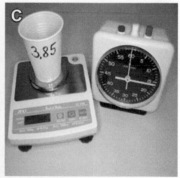

Fig. 6. Collection of whole saliva. (*A*) Sialometry requires a balance with 2 digits precision, a clock or timer, and a plastic cup. (*B*) The patient is seated comfortably in a chair and is instructed to keep the head tilted slightly forward, the mouth slightly open, the eyes open, and to minimize orofacial movements and to avoid swallowing of saliva during the collection process. The procedure should take place in a quiet room, where the patient can sit alone. The resting whole saliva flow rate is measured over a 15-minute period, during which the patient allows the saliva to accumulate in the floor of the mouth and then lets it drain into the preweighed plastic cup. The stimulated whole saliva flow rate is measured over a 5-minute period, during which the patient chews a piece of paraffin wax (neutral taste) with their own normal chewing frequency or stimulated by a 2% citric acid solution applied to the lateral borders of the tongue with a cotton applicator every 30 seconds, and spits the saliva into a preweighed plastic cup with a regular interval of 1 minute. (*C*) After the saliva collection, the plastic cup is weighed, including the collected saliva, and the weight of the plastic cup is subtracted, and divided by the collection time (ie, 15 minutes for the unstimulated and 5 minutes for the stimulated sialometry, respectively). Because 1 g is considered equivalent to 1 mL saliva, the flow rate is given in mL/min.[17]

then actively spit into the collected vessel every minute. The gustatory method uses a 2% (w/v) solution of citric acid to stimulate flow. The solution is applied to the lateral borders of the tongue with a cotton applicator every 30 seconds for 5 minutes. As with the chewing method, the saliva is expectorated into the collecting vessel every minute. The citric acid solution may be prepared and obtained from a local pharmacist.

Collection of Parotid Saliva

Parotid saliva is easy to collect. The orifice of the parotid gland is accessible for cannulation, but usually, a (modified) Lashley or Carlsson-Crittenden cup is used (**Fig. 7**). It is an easy procedure, which can be performed by even minimally trained personnel. The Lashley cup is a bichambered device, which measures about 2 cm in diameter. The inner chamber is placed directly over the orifice of the Stensen duct and connected, via plastic tubing, to a (graduated) test tube. The outer chamber is attached to a rubber bulb or a suction device via plastic tubing and is secured to the mucosa by vacuum. Because even in healthy individuals, the flow rate of unstimulated parotid saliva is very low or even absent, parotid saliva is usually collected under stimulated conditions. The most commonly applied

stimulus is a 2% to 4% (w/v) citric acid solution. This stimulus is applied to the lateral borders of the tongue at 30-second or 60-second intervals with a cotton swab. It is usually collected for 10 minutes. Burlage and colleagues[18] showed that there is a high correlation between flow rates from the left and right parotid glands (**Fig. 8**). This high correlation between flow rates of the left and right parotid glands may even be used as an internal check on reliability of a parotid saliva sample collected (flow rate of left parotid gland should be about the flow rate of the right parotid gland), unless a particular parotid gland show signs of inflammation or is involved in other salivary gland specific disease.

Collection of SM/SL Saliva

About 70% of the oral secretions stem from the combined SM/SL glands. Because of this situation, most studies show that the flow and composition of saliva obtained from the SM/SL glands is similar to that obtained with whole saliva. The suction method is generally used to obtain these secretions. In this technique, the Stenson ducts are blocked with either Lashley cups or cotton roles. This strategy allows SM/SL saliva to flow from the Warthin ducts and from the Bartholin and other SL ducts into the mouth. The saliva, which

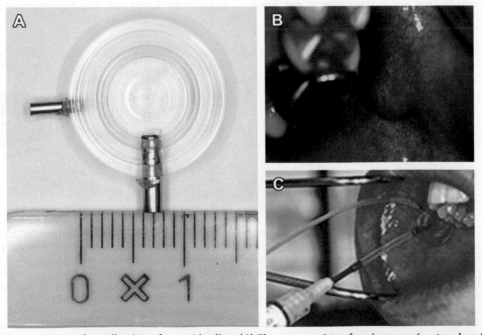

Fig. 7. The Lashley cup for collection of parotid saliva. (*A*) The cup consists of an inner and outer chamber. The inner chamber serves as the collection chamber; the outer chamber is for suction (it can be produced in metal or in transparent polymethylmethacrylate; ruler unit: centimeters). (*B*) The orifice of the parotid (Stenson) duct in the cheek. The cup is placed over this orifice. (*C*) The cup in place over the orifice of the parotid duct. The flow of parotid saliva is clearly visible in the inner chamber.

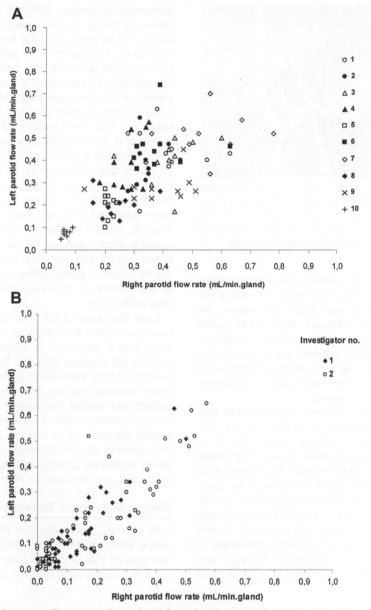

Fig. 8. Correlation between flow rates from the left and right parotid glands. Note the wide spread for the higher rates (*A*), the clustering of the flow rates for the lower secretion rates (*B*), and good agreement between the investigators. (*A*) Healthy volunteers. (*B*) Patients with SS. (*Reprinted from* Burlage FR, Pijpe J, Coppes RP, et al. Variability of flow rate when collecting stimulated human parotid saliva. Eur J Oral Sci 2005;113:386–90; with permission.)

accumulates on the floor of the mouth, can be aspirated with a syringe (**Fig. 9**), micropipette, or with gentle suction (see Wolff apparatus, **Fig. 10**). The SM/SL saliva can be collected in the resting or stimulated state. As with the parotid glands, a 2% to 4% (w/v) solution of citric acid is frequently used to stimulate flow. Mixing of the acid solution applied to the tongue with the SM/SL saliva that is present on the floor of the mouth should be carefully avoided.

New Developments in the Application of Saliva as a Diagnostic Tool

Although stimulated SM/SL flow rate in combination with parotid sodium and chloride concentration has been suggested as a reliable diagnostic test for SS,[5] recent progress in proteomics and genomics has shown that the proteomic and genomic profile may be more sensitive and specific in diagnosing SS.[19] When compared with

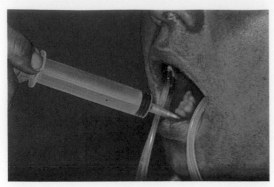

Fig. 9. The suction method for collection of SM/SL saliva. The orifices of the parotid ducts can be blocked with, for example, Lashley cups or cotton roles. The saliva collected in the floor of the mouth is now mainly SM/SL saliva and can be collected with a syringe.

healthy controls, 16 peptides present in whole saliva could be qualified as being differently expressed in patients with SS.[20] Moreover, the same investigators showed that whole saliva contains more informative proteins, peptides, and messenger RNA (mRNA) than parotid and SM/SL. This finding is not surprising because in whole saliva also contributions of, for example, serum exudates are present.

The next step is to further study whether biomarkers that are different between patients with SS and healthy individuals are specific for SS or are also commonly expressed in saliva of patients with other autoimmune diseases. As a first step, to look into the specificity of biomarkers for diagnosing SS, the SS proteomic/genomic profile was compared with that of patients with systemic lupus erythematosus (SLE) (all non-sSS). It was shown that 3 protein biomarkers (cathepsin D, α-enolase, and β$_2$-microglobulin [B2M]), and 3 mRNA biomarkers (myeloid cell nuclear

differentiation antigen [MNDA], guanylate binding protein 2 [GIP2], and the low-affinity IIIb receptor for the Fc fragment of IgG) were all significantly increased in patients with pSS compared with both patients with SLE and healthy controls. The combination of cathepsin D, α-enolase, and B2M yielded a receiver operating characteristic (ROC) value of 99% in distinguishing pSS from healthy controls. The combination of protein marker, B2M, and the mRNA biomarkers MNDA and GIP2, reached an ROC of 95% in discriminating pSS from SLE.[21,22] As soon as a definitive, highly sensitive and highly specific set of markers for diagnosing SS has been developed and has been validated in large, well-conducted clinical studies, this set of markers can be incorporated in point-of-care assays for use in daily practice. When such a point-of-care assay is available, it will be easier to screen patients for SS in the office of the dentist or physician, thus enabling early diagnosis of SS.

Early diagnosis of SS is of utmost importance, because intervention therapy with biologics may be a fruitful approach in patients with early SS or high SS disease activity. Proteomic/genomic analysis of pSS, followed by gene ontology or functional pathway analysis, may also show molecular targets and related pathways associated with the disease pathogenesis. These activated pathways in pSS provide further insights into the molecular mechanisms of the disease, and the identified genes represent promising targets for diagnosis, prognosis, and therapeutic intervention.[23]

Diagnostic Imaging Techniques

Until recently, it was obvious that magnetic resonance imaging (MRI) and ultrasonography (US) had proved their value as diagnostic instruments in SS, but sialography remains the best performing

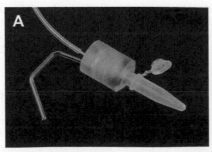
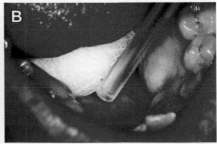

Fig. 10. SM/SL saliva collecting device (Wolff apparatus). (*A*) Two lengths of tubing, one for saliva collection (*left*) and the other for suction (*right*), are connected to the top of the buffering chamber. An additional hole is provided for manual suction control. A 1.5-mL centrifuge tube (for saliva storage) is attached to the bottom of the chamber. (*B*) Use of the SM/SL saliva collection device on gauze-covered SM/SL duct openings. (*Data from* Wolff A, Begleiter A, Moskona D. A novel system of human submandibular/sublingual saliva collection. J Dent Res 1997;76:1782–6.)

Table 4
Influence of conditions on salivary gland function. The 3 most important causes of a reduced salivary gland function are drugs, SS, and head and neck radiotherapy

	Flow Rate	Changed Composition	Xerostomia
Drugs			
Secretogogues	↑	±	−
Xerogenic drugs	↓	+	+
SS	↓	+	+
Head and neck radiotherapy	↓	+	+
Chronic inflammatory connective tissue diseases			
Scleroderma	↓	?	+
Mixed connective tissue disease	↓	?	+
Chronic inflammatory bowel diseases			
Crohn disease	→	+	+
Ulcerative colitis	→	+	−
Celiac disease	→	+	−
Autoimmune liver diseases	↓	?	+
Musculoskeletal disorders			
Fibromyalgia	↓	?	+
Chronic fatigue syndrome	↓	?	+
Amyloidosis	↓	?	+
Endocrine disorders			
Diabetes mellitus	↓	±	+
Hyperthyroidism	↑	+	−
Hypothyroidism	↓	?	+
Cushing syndrome	→	+	−
Addison disease	→	+	−
Neurologic disorders			
Central nervous system trauma	↓	?	?
Cerebral palsy	↓	+	?
Bell palsy	↓	+	?
Parkinson disease	↓	+	+
Alzheimer disease	↓	+	+
Holmes-Adie syndrome	↓	?	+
Burning mouth syndrome	→	+	+
Infectious diseases			
Epidemic parotitis	?	?	?
Human immunodeficiency virus/AIDS	↓	±	+
Hepatitis C virus	↓	?	+
Epstein-Barr virus	?	?	?
Tuberculosis	?	?	?
Local bacterial salivary gland infections	↓	+	?
Genetic disorders			
Salivary gland aplasia	↓	?	?
Cystic fibrosis	↓	+	?
Ectodermal dysplasia	↓	+	−
Prader-Willi syndrome	↓	+	?

(continued on next page)

Table 4
(continued)

	Flow Rate	Changed Composition	Xerostomia
Metabolic disturbances			
Water and salt balance	↓	+	+
Sodium retention syndrome	↓	+	+
Malnutrition	↓	+	+
Eating disorders			
Bulimia nervosa	↓	±	+
Anorexia nervosa	↓	+	+
Cancer-associated disturbances			
Chemotherapy	↓	±	+
Graft-versus-host disease	↓	+	+
Advanced cancer/terminally ill patients	↓	?	+

Abbreviations: ↓, decreased flow rate; ↑, increased flow rate; →, unchanged flow rate; +, yes; −, no; ±, differing results; ?, possibly affected/awaiting clinical studies.

Adapted from Jensen SB, Pedersen AM, Nauntofte B. The causes of dry mouth: a broad panoply. Other causes of dry mouth: the list is endless. In: Sreebny LM, Vissink A, editors. Dry mouth–the malevolent symptom: a clinical guide. 1st edition. Ames (IA): Wiley-Blackwell; 2010. p. 158–81.

diagnostic imaging technique in SS, with accuracy still higher than MRI and US.[24] However, US is rapidly keeping up with the sensitivity and specificity of sialography and MRI-sialography in diagnosing SS. Scintigraphy, although part of the American-European criteria for SS, scored poor when compared with sialography, MRI, and US. Moreover, when deciding which imaging technique to use in the diagnosis of SS, besides the diagnostic accuracy, the clinical usefulness, the applicability, the costs, and the invasiveness of the tests should be considered. Most studies on sialography, US, and MRI report high likelihood ratios (LR≥5), which indicates clinical usefulness. Sialography is a relatively quick procedure (<15 minutes), with low morbidity. However, it does involve exposure to ionizing radiation and infusion of iodized contrast fluid into the salivary gland. Furthermore, pain and swelling may occur after sialography, retention of contrast liquid may occur when an oil-based fluid is used, and the use of iodinated contrast material is contraindicated in patients with known iodine sensitivity. Another drawback of sialography is that the correct interpretation of the images requires expertise. However, the problem of pain and swelling is relative, because after a few days, pain and swelling often decrease to less than baseline level, a reason why parotid sialography is occasionally applied as a therapeutic approach in patients with persisting glandular pain and swelling. Also, retention of the contrast material is more a coincidence than a cause of further symptoms in the patient. Both

MRI and in particular US are considered biologically harmless, but are not yet included in the American-European Consensus Group (AECG) and American College of Rheumatology (ACR) criteria for SS.[6,25–27]

With regard to US, recently, many studies have been performed to assess the value of US in diagnosing SS. Cornec and colleagues[28] showed that adding US to the AECG criteria increased the sensitivity of AECG criteria for pSS from 78% to 87% and retained specificity. US seems to be a valid alternative (or even replacement) to sialography and salivary gland scintigraphy in the AECG criteria. Thus, US is a promising addition to the AECG criteria, and should also be tested in the ACR criteria. US and other noninvasive techniques should be extensively tested in the diagnostic setting, preferably to replace or limit the use of lip biopsy. US is likely to gain a place in monitoring disease activity and disease progression.[26]

How to Assess Xerostomia?

There are many causes of dry mouth (**Table 4**). Many of them can be rapidly ruled out by a systematic evaluation of the patient's medical history, by the findings obtained in the clinical examination, and by information obtained from laboratory tests (**Fig. 11**). For some patients, the initial complaint may solely be dry mouth. Others may report additional symptoms that accompany it. Virtually all of them bemoan the decrease in the quality of their lives since the advent of oral dryness.

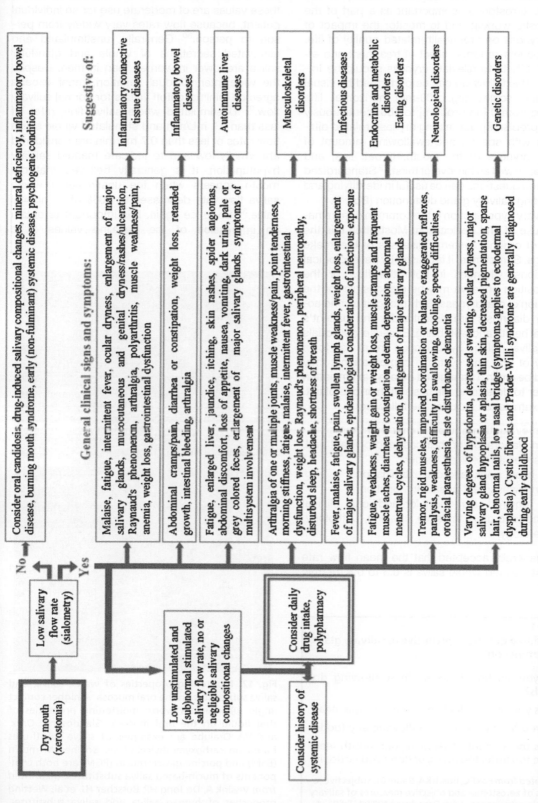

Fig. 11. Flow diagram for diagnosis of systemic diseases/conditions as causes of dry mouth. (*From* Jensen SB, Pedersen AM, Nauntofte B. The causes of dry mouth: a broad panoply. Other causes of dry mouth: the list is endless. In: Sreebny LM, Vissink A, editors. Dry mouth–the malevolent symptom: a clinical guide. 1st edition. Ames (IA): Wiley-Blackwell; 2010. p. 158–81; with permission.)

Assessment of the subjective feeling of dry mouth, xerostomia, is important as a part of the diagnostic workup and to monitor the impact of oral dryness on oral health-related quality of life. Also, patient-reported effect of treatment and effect of efforts to alleviate dryness should be followed. This follow-up can be performed by visual analogue scales (eg, 100-mm horizontal line ranging from 0 [no problem] to 100 [continuously major problems]) addressing dryness-related difficulties with speech and swallowing, amount of saliva, dryness of the mouth, throat, lips, and tongue, as well as the level of thirst.[29] Standardized validated questions can be useful in identifying and predicting salivary gland dysfunction (**Box 1**).[14]

Salivary hypofunction is the common denominator cause of oral desiccation. Most often it is the result of organic systemic diseases or the intake of drugs. Sometimes, it is caused by psychological conditions. Changes in both the flow or the composition of saliva may be responsible for the induction of oral dryness. Early recognition and accurate diagnosis are essential for the patient's general health and well-being. Because individuals with salivary gland hypofunction are at risk for a variety of oral and systemic complications, they should be given a careful and detailed examination in order to determine the basis of their complaint. This examination includes the following:

- An evaluation of the patient's symptoms
- An elaboration of their past and present oral, as well as medical, history
- A head, neck, and oral examination
- An assessment of salivary function
- If required, a request for additional clinical and laboratory tests (eg, imaging, pathology, serology)

It is generally accepted that the mean flow rate of unstimulated whole saliva is 0.3 to 0.4 mL/min

and of stimulated saliva, 1 to 2 mL/min. However, these values are of moderate use for an individual patient, because flow rates vary widely from person to person.[30] Generally, unstimulated and stimulated secretions of whole and glandular saliva are lower in women than in men. Despite the wide interindividual variation, most experts agree on minimal cutoff values for normal salivary flow.[31] Unstimulated whole saliva flow rates of less than 0.1 mL/min and stimulated whole saliva flow rates of less than 0.7 mL/min are considered abnormally low and to indicate marked salivary hypofunction. It is generally believed that dry mouth appears when the unstimulated whole saliva flow rate decreases to 50% of its normal value.[32] So, once again, it is important to obtain an impression of the baseline values of a

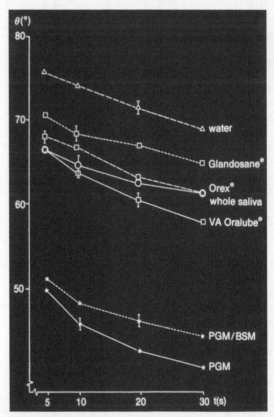

Fig. 12. Moistening properties of water, saliva, and saliva substitutes on the oral mucosa. A higher contact angle (θ) indicates worse moistening properties of that liquid on the oral mucosa. Glandosane, Orex, and VA Oralube are examples of saliva substitutes based on carboxymethylcellulose. Bovine SM mucin (BSM) and porcine gastric mucin (PGM) are both components of mucin-based saliva substitutes. (*Reprinted from* Vissink A, De Jong HP, Busscher HJ, et al. Wetting properties of human saliva and saliva substitutes. J Dent Res 1986;65:1121–4; with permission.)

Box 1
Validated questions predictive of salivary gland hypofunction

Do you sip liquids to aid in swallowing dry foods?

Does your mouth feel dry when eating a meal?

Do you have difficulties swallowing any foods?

Does the amount of saliva in your mouth seem to be too little, too much, or don't you notice it?

Adapted from Fox PC, Busch KA, Baum BJ. Subjective reports of xerostomia and objective measures of salivary gland performance. J Am Dent Assoc 1987;115:581–4.

Table 5
Short Form (SF)-36 scores for patients with SS and the general Dutch population

SF-36 Scales and Summary Scores	GDP (n = 195)	RSS (n = 195)	P Value (RSS vs GDP)	pSS (n = 154)	sSS (n = 41)	P Value (pSS vs sSS)
Physical functioning	74.8 ± 25.8	59.2 ± 26.0	.000	62.0 ± 25.1	48.9 ± 27.0	.004
Physical role functioning	70.3 ± 36.3	41.0 ± 42.9	.000	44.0 ± 42.7	29.1 ± 41.9	.058
Bodily pain	68.7 ± 25.6	64.7 ± 24.4	.136	68.0 ± 23.0	52.1 ± 25.7	.000
General health	65.7 ± 21.5	40.3 ± 18.2	.000	41.9 ± 18.4	34.2 ± 16.3	.018
Vitality	63.8 ± 21.0	45.2 ± 20.1	.000	46.0 ± 20.4	42.0 ± 18.9	.266
Social functioning	81.3 ± 25.6	63.1 ± 26.2	.000	64.5 ± 26.6	57.9 ± 24.5	.152
Emotional role functioning	79.7 ± 34.4	70.0 ± 41.4	.005	71.5 ± 41.5	63.9 ± 40.9	.324
Mental health	73.3 ± 19.0	70.3 ± 18.4	.055	70.6 ± 18.9	69.0 ± 16.8	.627
PCS	73.0 ± 24.6	51.7 ± 23.7	.000	53.3 ± 23.6	44.7 ± 23.2	.055
MCS	74.5 ± 21.1	63.3 ± 21.2	.000	64.0 ± 21.2	60.5 ± 21.4	.385

Values are given as mean ± standard deviation.
Abbreviations: GDP, general Dutch population; MCS, mental composite score; PCS, physical component summary score; RSS, all responding patients with SS.
Adapted from Meijer JM, Meiners PM, Huddleston Slater JJ, et al. Health-related quality of life, employment and disability in patients with Sjögren's syndrome. Rheumatology (Oxford) 2009;48:1077–82; with permission.

particular patient, because in some patients, the oral mucosa may appear moist on clinical inspection, but the patients still complain of oral dryness. In such cases, it might be useful to assess the flow of parotid and SM saliva. Patients in whom the contribution of the parotid glands is much higher than that of the SM glands might complain about oral dryness, because the water-like parotid saliva is a less effective moistener of the oral mucosa than the more viscous SM saliva (**Fig. 12**).[33]

IMPACT OF SS ON QUALITY OF LIFE

SS is known to affect patients' physical, psychological, and social functioning, but the impact of SS on health-related quality of life (HR-QOL), employment, and disability has not been studied extensively. Meijer and colleagues[34] showed that SS has a large impact on HR-QOL, employment, and disability, as reflected by lower Short Form 36 scores and employment rates, and higher disability rates when compared with the general Dutch population (**Table 5**). Further, analysis of HR-QOL revealed that patients with sSS were more limited in physical activities than patients with pSS, but did not differ in socioeconomic status, delay in diagnosis and untreated or undiagnosed depression.[35] Although the results were obtained from a Dutch cohort of patients with SS, the striking differences in HR-QOL, employment, and disability suggest that the results of that study are not limited to the Dutch population,

but probably are generally applicable to patients with SS when compared with healthy individuals. Meijer and colleagues found fatigue to be an important explanatory variable for reduced physical and mental HR QOL. This finding is in agreement with other studies.[36–38]

REFERENCES

1. Veerman EC, van den Keybus PA, Vissink A, et al. Human glandular salivas: their separate collection and analysis. Eur J Oral Sci 1996;104:346–52.
2. Nieuw Amerongen AV, Bolscher JG, Veerman EC. Salivary mucins: protective functions in relation to their diversity. Glycobiology 1995;5:733–40.
3. Tabak LA. In defense of the oral cavity: structure, biosynthesis, and function of salivary mucins. Annu Rev Physiol 1995;57:547–64.
4. DiSabato-Mordarski T, Kleinberg I. Measurement and comparison of the residual saliva on various oral mucosal and dentition surfaces in humans. Arch Oral Biol 1996;41:655–65.
5. Kalk WW, Vissink A, Spijkervet FK, et al. Sialometry and sialochemistry: diagnostic tools for Sjögren's syndrome. Ann Rheum Dis 2001;60:1110–6.
6. Vitali C, Bombardieri S, Jonsson R, et al. Classification criteria for Sjögren's syndrome: a revised version of the European criteria proposed by the American-European Consensus Group. Ann Rheum Dis 2002;61:554–8.
7. Pijpe J, Kalk WW, Bootsma H, et al. Progression of salivary gland dysfunction in patients with Sjögren's syndrome. Ann Rheum Dis 2007;66:107–12.

8. Pijpe J, Meijer JM, Bootsma H, et al. Clinical and histologic evidence of salivary gland restoration supports the efficacy of rituximab treatment in Sjögren's syndrome. Arthritis Rheum 2009;60:3251–6.

9. Pijpe J, van Imhoff GW, Spijkervet FK, et al. Rituximab treatment in patients with primary Sjögren's syndrome: an open-label phase II study. Arthritis Rheum 2005;52:2740–50.

10. Hansen A, Lipsky PE, Dorner T. Immunopathogenesis of primary Sjögren's syndrome: implications for disease management and therapy. Curr Opin Rheumatol 2005;17:558–65.

11. Nguyen CQ, Hu MH, Li Y, et al. Salivary gland tissue expression of interleukin-23 and interleukin-17 in Sjögren's syndrome: findings in humans and mice. Arthritis Rheum 2008;58:734–43.

12. Pijpe J, van Imhoff GW, Vissink A, et al. Changes in salivary gland immunohistology and function after rituximab monotherapy in a patient with Sjögren's syndrome and associated MALT lymphoma. Ann Rheum Dis 2005;64:958–60.

13. Youinou P, Devauchelle V, Hutin P, et al. A conspicuous role for B cells In Sjögren's syndrome. Clin Rev Allergy Immunol 2007;32:231–7.

14. Fox PC, Busch KA, Baum BJ. Subjective reports of xerostomia and objective measures of salivary gland performance. J Am Dent Assoc 1987;115:581–4.

15. Sreebny LM, Vissink A. Sialometry: the measure of things, with ease and reliability. In: Sreebny LM, Vissink A, editors. Dry mouth–the malevolent symptom: a clinical guide. 1st edition. Ames (IA): Wiley-Blackwell; 2010. p. 64–76.

16. Vissink A, Wolff A, Veerman ECI. Saliva collectors. In: Wong DT, editor. Saliva diagnostics. Ames (IA): Wiley-Blackwell; 2008. p. 37–59.

17. Navazesh M, Christensen CM. A comparison of whole mouth resting and stimulated salivary measurement procedures. J Dent Res 1982;61:1158–62.

18. Burlage FR, Pijpe J, Coppes RP, et al. Variability of flow rate when collecting stimulated human parotid saliva. Eur J Oral Sci 2005;113:386–90.

19. Vissink A, Bootsma H, Kroese FG, et al. How to assess treatment efficacy in Sjögren's syndrome? Curr Opin Rheumatol 2012;24:281–9.

20. Hu S, Wang J, Meijer J, et al. Salivary proteomic and genomic biomarkers for primary Sjögren's syndrome. Arthritis Rheum 2007;56:3588–600.

21. Hu S, Vissink A, Arellano M, et al. Identification of autoantibody biomarkers for primary Sjögren's syndrome using protein microarrays. Proteomics 2011;11:1499–507.

22. Hu S, Gao K, Pollard R, et al. Preclinical validation of salivary biomarkers for primary Sjögren's syndrome. Arthritis Care Res (Hoboken) 2010;62:1633–8.

23. Hu S, Zhou M, Jiang J, et al. Systems biology analysis of Sjögren's syndrome and mucosa-associated lymphoid tissue lymphoma in parotid glands. Arthritis Rheum 2009;60:81–92.

24. Takagi Y, Kimura Y, Nakamura H, et al. Salivary gland ultrasonography: can it be an alternative to sialography as an imaging modality for Sjögren's syndrome? Ann Rheum Dis 2010;69:1321–4.

25. Vitali C, Bootsma H, Bowman SJ, et al. Classification criteria for Sjögren's syndrome: we actually need to definitively resolve the long debate on the issue. Ann Rheum Dis 2013;72:476–8.

26. Bootsma H, Spijkervet FK, Kroese FG, et al. Toward new classification criteria for Sjögren's syndrome? Arthritis Rheum 2013;65:21–3.

27. Shiboski SC, Shiboski CH, Criswell L, et al. American College of Rheumatology classification criteria for Sjögren's syndrome: a data-driven, expert consensus approach in the Sjögren's International Collaborative Clinical Alliance cohort. Arthritis Care Res (Hoboken) 2012;64:475–87.

28. Cornec D, Jousse-Joulin S, Pers JO, et al. Contribution of salivary gland ultrasonography to the diagnosis of Sjögren's syndrome: toward new diagnostic criteria? Arthritis Rheum 2013;65:216–25.

29. Pai S, Ghezzi EM, Ship JA. Development of a visual analogue scale questionnaire for subjective assessment of salivary dysfunction. Oral Surg Oral Med Oral Pathol Oral Radiol Endod 2001;91:311–6.

30. Ship JA, Fox PC, Baum BJ. How much saliva is enough? 'Normal' function defined. J Am Dent Assoc 1991;122:63–9.

31. Sreebny LM. Saliva in health and disease: an appraisal and update. Int Dent J 2000;50:140–61.

32. Dawes C. Physiological factors affecting salivary flow rate, oral sugar clearance, and the sensation of dry mouth in man. J Dent Res 1987;(66 Spec No):648–53.

33. Vissink A, De Jong HP, Busscher HJ, et al. Wetting properties of human saliva and saliva substitutes. J Dent Res 1986;65:1121–4.

34. Meijer JM, Meiners PM, Huddleston Slater JJ, et al. Health-related quality of life, employment and disability in patients with Sjögren's syndrome. Rheumatology (Oxford) 2009;48:1077–82.

35. Belenguer R, Ramos-Casals M, Brito-Zeron P, et al. Influence of clinical and immunological parameters on the health-related quality of life of patients with primary Sjögren's syndrome. Clin Exp Rheumatol 2005;23:351–6.

36. Barendregt PJ, Visser MR, Smets EM, et al. Fatigue in primary Sjögren's syndrome. Ann Rheum Dis 1998;57:291–5.

37. Bjerrum K, Prause JU. Primary Sjögren's syndrome: a subjective description of the disease. Clin Exp Rheumatol 1990;8:283–8.

38. Tensing EK, Solovieva SA, Tervahartiala T, et al. Fatigue and health profile in sicca syndrome of

Sjögren's and non-Sjögren's syndrome origin. Clin Exp Rheumatol 2001;19:313–6.

39. Schneyer LH. Source of resting total mixed saliva of man. J Appl Physiol 1956;9:79–81.

40. Dawes C, Wood CM. The contribution of oral minor mucous gland secretions to the volume of whole saliva in man. Arch Oral Biol 1973;18: 337–42.

41. Dawes C, Ong BY. Circadian rhythms in the flow rate and proportional contribution of parotid to whole saliva volume in man. Arch Oral Biol 1973;18: 1145–53.

Oral Complications of Sjögren's Syndrome

Joel J. Napeñas, DDS, FDS RCS(Ed)[a,b,*],
Tanya S. Rouleau, DMD, FDS RCS(Ed)[b]

KEYWORDS

- Sjögren's syndrome • Caries • Periodontal disease • Burning mouth • Candidiasis

KEY POINTS

- A consensus exists that patients with Sjögren's syndrome are more prone to dental caries, with decay often occurring in areas that are not usually caries-prone.
- Although it is presumed that decreased salivary flow may lead to increases in periodontal disease, there is no increase in incidence and severity in patients with Sjögren's syndrome.
- Both intraoral and extraoral *Candida* infections are often found in patients with Sjögren's syndrome.
- Oral lesions may be found in patients with Sjögren's syndrome because of poor lubrication and subsequent trauma from dentures, food, or mucosal tissue contact with teeth.
- There is an increase in burning mouth, glossodynia, and neuropathies in patients with Sjögren's syndrome; however, there is no increased incidence of temporomandibular disorders. There is conflicting evidence with respect to migraine, tension-type, and other headache disorders.
- Patients with Sjögren's syndrome may complain of difficulty with speech, taste, and swallowing. They may also have swollen salivary glands and complaints of reflux disease.

INTRODUCTION

Most orofacial manifestations of Sjögren's syndrome (SS) are primarily a result of salivary gland hypofunction, which can be measured in an objective manner. Hyposalivation may lead to a subjective complaint of xerostomia. Treatment measures are usually aimed at alleviating symptoms. Furthermore, other nonsalivary gland associated complications have been implicated or associated with SS.

Many of the orofacial manifestations reported are encountered in patients with SS; however, these can also be seen in patients with hyposalivation from other etiologies (ie, systemic medications, head and neck radiation, and other systemic diseases). Additionally, when oral manifestations are studied in an SS population, there are a wide range of criteria for SS diagnosis, and not a clear delineation between patients with primary SS (pSS) or secondary SS. This article reviews those suspected or documented oral complications of SS (**Box 1**).

SALIVA FUNCTION

The three paired major salivary glands (parotid, submandibular, and sublingual) are responsible for 90% of oral secretions,[1] with the average adult producing 0.4 mL of saliva per minute, or 1.5 L per day.[2] Hyposalivation is a hallmark of SS, and diminished saliva is detrimental to function, but

Funding Sources: Nil.
Conflict of Interest: Nil.

[a] Division of Oral Medicine and Radiology, Schulich School of Medicine and Dentistry, Western University, Dental Sciences Building, London, Ontario N6A 5C1, Canada; [b] Department of Oral Medicine, Carolinas Medical Center, PO Box 32861, Charlotte, NC 28232, USA
* Corresponding author. Division of Oral Medicine and Radiology, Schulich School of Medicine and Dentistry, Western University, Dental Sciences Building, London, Ontario N6A 5C1, Canada.
E-mail address: joel.napenas@schulich.uwo.ca

Box 1
Implicated orofacial complications of Sjögren's syndrome (other than xerostomia and/or salivary hypofunction)

Evidence supporting association with Sjögren's syndrome

   Dental caries

   Candidiasis

   Burning mouth

   Peripheral neuropathies

   Glossodynia

   Dysphagia

   Dysgeusia

   Trouble speaking

   Oral lesions

   Swollen salivary glands

   Gastroesophageal reflux disease

Conflicting evidence

   Periodontal disease

   Migraine headaches

   Tension-type headaches

No evidence showing association with Sjögren's syndrome

   Temporomandibular disorders

also to quality of life. Saliva plays an important role in facilitating speech, providing lubrication, buffering, remineralizing enamel, assisting in taste, formation of food bolus, initiating digestion, and aiding in host defenses against infection.[1,3] Oral balance is maintained by the balance of salivary components including proteins, glycoproteins, enzymes, electrolytes, and small organic molecules.[1]

Salivary proteins serve many essential functions. Lysozyme, histatins, and defensins are antimicrobial; proline-rich proteins help in enamel pellicle formation and enamel surface mineralization; statherin facilitates enamel remineralization by concentrating calcium and phosphate and may inhibit calculus formation; and mucins allow lubrication.[4]

CHANGES IN ORAL MICROFLORA

Decreased salivary flow rates, such as those seen in SS, result in a modified oral microbial plaque composition.[5] Although it has been found that total bacterial counts[6] and salivary counts of periodontopathogenic microorganisms *Fusobacterium nucleatum* and *Prevotella intermedia/nigriscens*

were similar in patients with SS and control subjects,[7] increased number and frequency of cariogenic microorganisms *Lactobacillus* spp, and *Streptococcus mutans* in supragingival plaque, and *Candida albicans* were found in patients with SS.[8] The oral flora changes are attributed to the change in salivary flow and the physical changes attributed to higher likelihood of dental restorations in these patients. Celenligil and colleagues[9] examined serum antibody responses to a group of gram-positive and -negative bacteria in the plaque of patients with SS. They demonstrated that there were significantly higher antibody levels to *Actinobacillus actinomycetemcomitans* and *Porphyromonas gingivalis* in SS compared with control subjects; however, there were significantly lower levels of antibody levels to *Streptococcus oralis*. This illustrated a normal host immune response to the presumed increased bacterial colonization of periodontal pathogens in patients with SS, and is in line with other studies showing decreased colonization of *S oralis* in patients with xerostomia.[10]

DENTAL MANIFESTATIONS
Caries

Dental caries development is a complex interplay between dietary factors, time, substrate, and bacteria. Characteristics of saliva are also important, including flow, composition, buffer and sugar clearance capacity, fluoride concentration, and more.[11] Xerostomia results in a decrease in secretory IgA, an antibody responsible for mucosal immunity, thereby weakening the defense system against dental caries.[2] Individuals with SS have a much lower pH and buffer capacity, with Mathews and coworkers[1] reporting this specifically in relation to the parotid gland when comparing findings with normal control subjects. Phosphate, bicarbonate, and protein are responsible for the buffering capacity of saliva. A small pH drop can cause dental caries or enamel erosion.[12] Additionally, lessened salivary flow (specifically unstimulated)[13] has been associated with increased time for sugar clearance and therefore increased levels of dental decay.[14]

Dental plaque, made up of a complex array of bacteria, forms a biofilm that adheres to teeth surfaces and provides a reservoir for pathogenic microbes.[15] Persons with SS have been reported to have higher numbers of cariogenic and acidophilic microorganisms compared with control subjects.[3,6,12,16,17] Specifically, low saliva flow has been associated with high bacterial levels of *Lactobacillus acidophilus* and *S mutans*, which has been postulated to explain the increased caries rate in patients with SS.[6]

The mechanical forces of salivary flow and the action of the tongue, cheeks, and lips rubbing the teeth act to dislodge bacteria from the tooth surfaces and oral cavity.[18] Patients with SS often have food pocketing in vestibules and around teeth resulting from poor lubrication and lack of mechanical action.

Often dental caries occurs at tooth-restoration interfaces and at locations that are not usually caries-prone, such as root, buccal/facial, and incisal/cuspal surfaces (**Fig. 1**).[3,11,19,20] Dental decay may lead to tooth loss, and those with SS have often been reported with more or earlier tooth loss, or a higher Decayed, Missing, Filled Teeth (DMFT) index compared with the general population.[11] Christensen and colleagues[21] studied patients with pSS and compared them with age-matched control subjects, finding that those with pSS had more teeth removed, a higher DMFT index, more trouble with their teeth in their lifetime, more dental visits, and higher dental costs compared with control subjects. Fox and colleagues[22] similarly reported patients with pSS having a significantly greater number of dental visits, more decayed teeth, and more dental restorations in the preceding year, in comparison with control subjects.

Gingivitis/Periodontal Disease

Although the relationship between SS and dental caries is well established, there is equivocal literature concerning its effects on the periodontium.

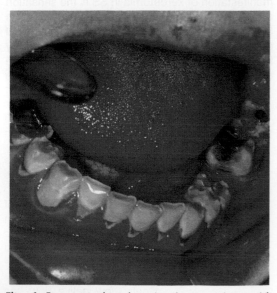

Fig. 1. Rampant dental caries in a patient with Sjögren's syndrome. Caries is noted at tooth-restoration interfaces, and at locations that are not usually caries-prone, such as root, facial, incisal, and cuspal surfaces.

Conceivably, the loss of saliva and its ability to prevent the formation of dental plaque may account for possible increases in calculus formation and periodontal disease. This is supported by studies on experimental animals that have shown that the removal of salivary glands significantly increased the incidence of periodontal disease[23]; however, a consistent relationship between amount of saliva and periodontal disease has not been observed in healthy individuals.[24] Although it has been shown that patients with SS have significantly lower levels of supragingival plaque than patients without SS with periodontitis and healthy control subjects,[25] other studies have shown that plaque index (PI) scores were increased in patients with SS with lower salivary flow rates.[26] Another hypothesis to suggest a link to periodontal disease includes immune dysfunction in SS, which may affect immune responses to bacterial challenges in the periodontium. Pers and colleagues[27] examined salivary levels of B-cell activating factor, which has been observed to be overexpressed in SS. They found that clinical parameters seen in periodontitis, including probing depths (PD), were associated with high levels of B-cell activating factor in saliva compared with control subjects, indicating its potential role in the pathogenesis of periodontal disease. Scardina and colleagues[28] found alterations in the interdental papilla microcirculation in patients with SS, suggesting that variation in vascular reactivity in SS may account for the impact of SS on the periodontium.

Conflicting evidence exists whether patients with SS are at increased risk for periodontal disease. One study found no risk for the development of periodontal disease[29] and multiple studies report no differences with regards to parameters measuring periodontal disease, which included PD, clinical attachment loss, and bleeding on probing.[30–36] However, several studies suggest otherwise. Najera and colleagues[37] found that although there was not an increased incidence of diagnosed periodontitis between patients with SS and control subjects, patients with SS had significantly higher PI scores, increased alveolar bone loss, and increased clinical attachment loss, in addition to a 2.2 times greater risk of developing periodontal disease. Of note, patients with SS engaged in more frequent oral hygiene habits than the control subjects. Among patients with SS, Celenligil and colleagues[9] also found increased PI scores in addition to sulcular bleeding and PD, whereas Pedersen and colleagues[38] reported higher PD. Differences in experimental design may account for the conflicting outcomes. In addition, therapeutic measures against SS (eg, nonsteroidal anti-inflammatory drugs, corticosteroids, antirheumatic drugs) may have an impact on the inflammatory response in periodontal disease.[26]

ORAL MUCOSAL MANIFESTATIONS
Fungal Infection

Persons with SS have an increased occurrence of fungal infections, with *C albicans* more frequent than the general population.[39,40] An inverse relationship between salivary flow rates (specifically a low stimulated flow)[40] and the level of *Candida* infection has been described by Tapper-Jones and colleagues.[41] This is secondary to decreased buffering capacity and salivary output, and the immunocompromised status of patients with SS.[1] Intraorally, *Candida* infection may present as erythematous mucosal lesions, denture stomatitis, and tongue fissuring (**Figs. 2** and **3**).[19] Chronic erythematous *Candida* infection is reported in 70% to 75% of patients with SS.[6,42] *Candida* colonization extraorally causes a dry, cracked, and erythematous appearance at the corners of the mouth.[1]

Oral Lesions

Saliva plays an important role in lubrication, preventing traumatic or frictional injury of the tongue, lips, and buccal mucosa. Additional frictional injury to the tissues lining the mouth can occur from eating foods that are sharp or rough, such as toast or chips (**Fig. 4**). Patients with xerostoma and patients with SS may have dry and cracked lips with peeling, sores of the oral mucosa, and tongue depapillation.[6,19,22,43] The tongue appearance of patients with SS has been described to look like

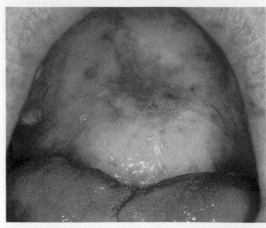

Fig. 3. Erythematous candidiasis on the hard palate of a patient with Sjögren's syndrome.

ground beef, with a desiccated, deeply fissured, and sticky appearance.[1,6]

With increased DMFT scores, some patients with SS experience partial or total edentulism. Dentures are oftentimes poorly tolerated because patients with xerostomia have reduced retention.[1,11] Traumatic lesions may result in the denture supporting tissues as they become fragile.[44,45]

OROFACIAL PAIN
Burning Mouth

Often accompanied by the most common oral manifestation of xerostomia in SS is the sensation of oral burning, or glossodynia.[46] Oral burning in SS is most likely attributed to secondary fungal infection as a result of the decreased salivary flow from SS (described previously),[44] and/or use of medications that impair salivary function. It is

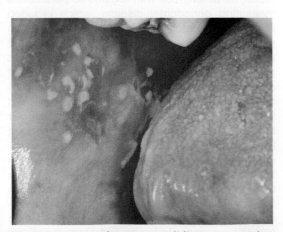

Fig. 2. Psuedomembranous candidiasis in a patient with Sjögren's syndrome. Although pseudomembranes were widespread in this patient's mouth, it was refractory to initial topical antifungal therapy.

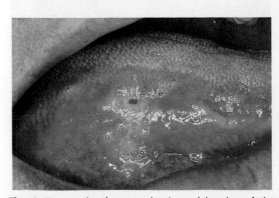

Fig. 4. Traumatic ulcer on the lateral border of the tongue of a patient with Sjögren's syndrome. Patient had a history of recurrent ulcerations for many years, attributed to lack of mucosal lubrication from decreased salivary flow.

conceivable that SS-associated neuropathies (described next) may also manifest as glossodynia and oral burning. Differential diagnoses of oral burning should also include anemia, allergies, oral lesions, and burning mouth syndrome.

Neurologic

The prevalence of peripheral nervous system manifestations in SS has been estimated to be in the range of 5% to 20%. However, the true prevalence has been controversial because of methodologic and clinical discrepancies that result in either overestimation or underestimation.[47] Most common are the symmetric distal sensory neuropathies[48]; however, sensorimotor neuropathies, autonomic neuropathies, and cranial neuropathies are also commonly found.[49] Small-fiber neuropathies present with the cardinal feature of excruciating burning pain, with subacute or chronic onset occurring over days to months, most commonly occurring in the upper and lower extremities. The most common cranial neuropathy in SS is trigeminal neuropathy, which typically occurs bilaterally, is progressive, and may be characterized by facial numbness or paresthesia with or without pain.[50] Sensory neuropathies are more common than motor dysfunction, with the facial nerve being the most commonly involved motor nerve.

Headaches

Gökçay and colleagues[51] found 78.1% of patients with pSS have headaches under the International Headache Society classification, which is higher than the prevalence of headaches among the general population. Among the diagnoses, migraine was the most common type (54%), followed by tension type headache (24.1%). A similar difference between patients with SS and control subjects was seen in a study by Pal and colleagues.[52] However, Tjensvoll and colleagues[53] found that the incidence of tension-type headaches was higher in patients with SS, but they did not have a higher incidence of migraines, and overall incidence of headaches. It is postulated that dysfunction of endothelial cells, which release factors involved in the pathogenesis of migraines, are also responsible in the pathogenesis of Raynaud phenomenon and antiphospholipid antibodies seen in patients with connective tissue disorders, such as SS.[48]

Temporomandibular Disorder

List and colleagues[54] performed a small study (N = 33) comparing the incidence of temporomandibular disorder (TMD) and related signs and symptoms in patients with SS, those diagnosed with TMD, and control subjects. The signs included mandibular range of motion, jaw joint sounds, and masticatory muscles that were tender to palpation. They found that the subjective, clinical, and radiographic signs of TMD are not more common in patients with pSS than in control subjects. Although the SS patient and TMD groups reported comparable levels of mandibular functioning related to speech and chewing ability, the SS group reported significantly greater interference with daily activities than the TMD group. This suggests that the effects of xerostomia are more debilitating than that of masticatory pain in patients with SS.

OTHER ORAL MANIFESTATIONS
Dysphagia/Dysguesia

Chewing, speaking, and swallowing are difficult as a result of intraoral dryness.[1,11,22] Swallowing food may require extra water intake to overcome swallowing difficulties.[11] Other subjective symptoms of oral dryness common to the SS patient population include sensitivity to flavorful foods, altered or diminished taste, oral pain, and coughing episodes or choking.[3,22]

Swollen Salivary Glands

Swollen salivary glands have been commonly reported in the SS patient population. The American European Consensus Criteria for diagnosis of SS has as one of its diagnostic components a question asking if patients have had swollen salivary glands in adulthood. Theander and colleagues[55] found salivary gland enlargement in 20% of their 484 patients investigated. Parotid gland swelling in particular has been reported to occur in 30% to 40% of patients with SS.[56] Sudden swelling of a single gland is suggestive of infection, with asymptomatic involvement of multiple glands with lymphadenopathy, of long-standing nature, being worrisome for lymphoma (discussed elsewhere in this issue).[22,57,58]

Gastroesophageal Reflux

Patients with SS have been found to have more esophageal dysmotility and symptoms of gastroesophageal reflux disease (GERD) than healthy individuals.[59] The potential for gastric acid contents to enter the mouth is associated with increased dental erosion.[60,61] Wan Nik and colleagues[62] found that patients with SS reported having an increased incidence of GERD-associated symptoms (heartburn, regurgitation) than control subjects, and had a significantly increased percentage of surfaces affecting the dentin with tooth wear. However, they did not find significant differences in tooth wear prevalence between patients with SS with and without symptoms of GERD.

SUMMARY

Most well-documented oral complications associated with SS (ie, infectious, such as dental caries and candidiasis; oral lesions; functional difficulties) are direct manifestations of decreased saliva in the oral cavity. In addition, there are several other conditions associated with this patient population (eg, swollen salivary glands, neuropathic pain, GERD). Consequently, management of these patients entails treatment of symptoms and prevention and treatment of infectious processes (discussed in the articles by Pinto as well as by Wu and Carsons elsewhere in this issue).

REFERENCES

1. Mathews SA, Kurien BT, Scofield RH. Oral manifestations of Sjögren's syndrome. J Dent Res 2008;87: 308–18.
2. Astor FC, Hanft KL, Ciocon JO. Xerostomia: a prevalent condition in the elderly. Ear Nose Throat J 1999;78:476–9.
3. Soto-Rojas AE, Kraus A. The oral side of Sjögren syndrome. Diagnosis and treatment. A review. Arch Med Res 2002;33:95–106.
4. Hsu SD, Dickinson DP, Qin H, et al. Green tea polyphenols reduce autoimmune symptoms in a murine model for human Sjogren's syndrome and protect human salivary acinar cells from TNF-alpha-induced cytotoxicity. Autoimmunity 2007; 40:138–47.
5. Marsh PD. Microbial ecology of dental plaque and its significance in health and disease. Adv Dent Res 1994;8:263–71.
6. Lundström IM, Lindström FD. Subjective and clinical oral symptoms in patients with primary Sjögren's syndrome. Clin Exp Rheumatol 1995;13: 725–31.
7. Almstahl A, Kroneld U, Tarkowski A, et al. Oral microbial flora in Sjögren's syndrome. J Rhematol 1999;26:110–4.
8. Leung KC, Leung WK, McMillan AS. Supra-gingival microbiota in Sjögren's syndrome. Clin Oral Invest 2007;11:415–23.
9. Celenligil H, Eratalay K, Kansu E, et al. Periodontal status and serum antibody responses to oral microorganisms in Sjögren's syndrome. J Periodontol 1998;69:571–7.
10. Hillman JD. Principles of microbial ecology and their application to xerostomia-associated opportunistic infections of the oral cavity. Adv Dent Res 1996;10:66–8.
11. González S, Sung H, Sepúlveda D, et al. Oral manifestations and their treatment in Sjögren's syndrome. Oral Dis 2013. http://dx.doi.org/10.1111/odi.12105. [Epub ahead of print].
12. Pedersen AM, Bardow A, Nauntofte B. Salivary changes and dental caries as potential oral markers of autoimmune salivary gland dysfunction in primary Sjogren's syndrome. BMC Clin Pathol 2005;5(1):4.
13. Bardow A, ten Cate JM, Nauntofte B, et al. Effect of unstimulated saliva flow rate on experimental root caries. Caries Res 2003;37:232–6.
14. Leone CW, Oppenheim FG. Physical and chemical aspects of saliva as indicators of risk for dental caries in humans. J Dent Educ 2001;65: 1054–62.
15. Paster BJ, Boches SK, Galvin JL, et al. Bacterial diversity in human subgingival plaque. J Bacteriol 2001;183:3770–83.
16. Sreebny L, Zhu WX. Whole saliva and the diagnosis of Sjögren's syndrome: an evaluation of patients who complain of dry mouth and dry eyes. Part 1: screening tests. Gerodontology 1996;13: 35–43.
17. Kolavic SA, Gibson G, al-Hashimi I, et al. The level of cariogenic micro-organisms in patients with Sjögren's syndrome. Spec Care Dentist 1997;17: 65–9.
18. Daniels TE, Fox PC. Salivary and oral components of Sjögren's syndrome. Rheum Dis Clin North Am 1992;18:571–89.
19. Mavragani CP, Moutsopoulos NM, Moutsopoulos HM. The management of Sjögren's syndrome. Nat Clin Pract Rheumatol 2006;2: 252–61.
20. Newbrun E. Current treatment modalities of oral problems of patients with Sjögren's syndrome: caries prevention. Adv Dent Res 1996; 10:29–34.
21. Christensen LB, Petersen PE, Thorn JJ, et al. Dental caries and dental health behavior of patients with primary Sjögren syndrome. Acta Odontol Scand 2001;59:116–20.
22. Fox PC, Bowman SJ, Segal B, et al. Oral involvement in primary Sjögren syndrome. J Am Dent Assoc 2008;139:1592–601.
23. Gupta OP, Blechman H, Stahl SS. The effects of desalivation on periodontal tissues of the Syrian hamster. Oral Surg Oral Med Oral Pathol 1960;13: 470–81.
24. Crow HC, Ship JA. Are gingival and periodontal conditions related to salivary gland flow rates in healthy individuals? J Am Dent Assoc 1995;126: 1514–20.
25. Socransky SS, Haffajee AD. Periodontal microbial ecology. Periodontol 2000 2005;38: 135–87.

26. Antoniazzi RP, Miranda LA, Zanatta FB, et al. Periodontal conditions of individuals with Sjögren's syndrome. J Periodontol 2009;80:429–35.

27. Pers JO, d'Arbonneau F, Devauchelle-Pensec V, et al. Is periodontal disease mediated by salivary BAFF in Sjögren's syndrome? Arthritis Rheum 2005;52:2411–4.

28. Scardina GA, Ruggieri A, Messina P. Periodontal disease and Sjögren syndrome: a possible correlation? Angiology 2010;6:289–93.

29. Pedersen AM, Reibel J, Nauntoffte B. Primary Sjögren's syndrome (pSS): subjective symptoms and salivary findings. J Oral Pathol Med 1999;287:303–11.

30. Ravald N, List T. Caries and periodontal conditions in patients with primary Sjögren's syndrome. Swed Dent J 1998;22:97–103.

31. Tseng CC. Periodontal status of patients with Sjögren's syndrome: a cross-sectional study. J Formos Med Assoc 1991;90:109–11.

32. Tervahrtiala T, Ingman T, Sorsa T, et al. Proteolytic enzymes as indicators of periodontal health in gingival crevicular fluid of patients with Sjögren's syndrome. Eur J Oral Sci 1995;103:11–6.

33. Boutsi EA, Paikos S, Dafni UG, et al. Dental and periodontal status of Sjögren's syndrome. J Clin Periodontol 2000;27:231–5.

34. Kuru B, McCullogh MJ, Yilmaz S, et al. Clinical and microbiological studies of periodontal disease in Sjögren's syndrome patients. J Clin Periodontol 2002;29:92–102.

35. Jorkjend L, Johansson A, Johansson AK, et al. Periodontitis, caries and salivary factors in Sjögren's syndrome patients compared to sex- and age-matched controls. J Oral Rehabil 2003;30:369–78.

36. Schiødt M, Christensen LB, Petersen PE, et al. Periodontal disease in primary Sjögren's syndrome. Oral Dis 2001;7:106–8.

37. Najera MP, Al-Hashimi I, Plemons JM, et al. Prevalence of periodontal disease in patients with Sjögren's syndrome. Oral Surg Oral Med Oral Pathol Oral Radiol Endod 1997;83:453–7.

38. Pedersen AM, Reibel J, Nordgarden H, et al. Primary Sjögren's syndrome: salivary gland function and clinical oral findings. Oral Dis 1999;5:128–38.

39. MacFarlane TW, Mason DK. Changes in the oral flora in Sjögren's syndrome. J Clin Pathol 1974;27:416–9.

40. Radfar L, Shea Y, Fischer SH, et al. Fungal load and candidiasis in Sjögren's syndrome. Oral Surg Oral Med Oral Pathol Oral Radiol Endod 2003;96:283–7.

41. Tapper-Jones L, Aldred M, Walker DM. Prevalence and intraoral distribution of Candida albicans in Sjögren's syndrome. J Clin Pathol 1980;33:282–7.

42. Soto-Rojas AE, Villa AR, Sifuentes-Osornio J, et al. Oral candidiasis and Sjögren's syndrome. J Rheumatol 1998;25:911–5.

43. Soto-Rojas AE, Villa AR, Sifuentes-Osornia J, et al. Oral manifestations in patients with Sjögren's syndrome. J Rheumatol 1998;25:906–10.

44. Ship JA. Diagnosing, managing, and preventing salivary gland disorders. Oral Dis 2002;8:77–89.

45. Cannon RD, Chaffin WL. Oral colonization by Candida albicans. Crit Rev Oral Biol Med 1999;10:359–83.

46. Al-Hashimi I, Khuder S, Haghighat N, et al. Frequency and predictive value of the clinical manifestations in Sjögren's syndrome. Diagnosis and treatment. A review. Arch Med Res 2002;33:95–106.

47. Birnbaum J. Peripheral nervous system manifestations of Sjögren's syndrome. Neurologist 2010;16:287–97.

48. Olney RK. Neuropathies associated with connective tissue disease. Semin Neurol 1998;18:63–72.

49. Mellgren SI, Conn DL, Stevens JC, et al. Peripheral neuropathy in primary Sjögren's syndrome. Neurology 1989;39:390–4.

50. Klasser GD, Blasubramaniam R, Epstein J. Topical review-connective tissue diseases: orofacial manifestations including pain. J Orofac Pain 2007;21:171–84.

51. Gökçay F, Öder G, Çelebisoy N, et al. Headache in primary Sjögren's syndrome: a prevalence study. Acta Neurol Scand 2008;118:189–92.

52. Pal B, Givson C, Passmore J, et al. A study of headaches and migraine in Sjögren's syndrome and other rheumatic disorders. Ann Rheum Dis 1989;48:312–6.

53. Tjensvoll AB, Harboe E, Göransson LG, et al. Headache in primary Sjögren's syndrome: a population-based retrospective cohort study. Eur J Neurol 2013;20:558–63.

54. List T, Stenström B, Lundström I, et al. TMD in patients with primary Sjögren syndrome: a comparison with temporomandibular clinic cases and controls. J Orofac Pain 1999;13:21–8.

55. Theander E, Manthorpe R, Jacobsson LT. Mortality and causes of death in primary Sjögren's syndrome: a prospective cohort study. Arthritis Rheum 2004;50:1262–9.

56. Pertovaara M, Korpela M, Uusitalo H, et al. Clinical follow up study of 87 patients with sicca symptoms (dryness of eyes or mouth, or both). Ann Rheum Dis 1999;58:423–7.

57. Freeman SR, Sheehan PZ, Thorpe MA, et al. Ear, nose, and throat manifestations of Sjögren's syndrome: retrospective review of a multidisciplinary clinic. J Otolaryngol 2005;34:20–4.

58. Harris NL. Lymphoid proliferations of the salivary glands. Am J Clin Pathol 1999;111:S94–103.

59. Mandl T, Ekberg O, Wollmer P, et al. Dysphagia and dysmotility of the pharynx and oesophagus in patients with primary Sjögren's syndrome. Scand J Rheumatol 2007;36:394–401.

60. Bartlett DW, Evans DF, Anggiansah A, et al. A study of the association between gastro-oesophageal reflux and palatal dental erosion. Br Dent J 1996;181: 125–32.

61. Pace F, Pallota S, Tonini M, et al. Systematic review: gastro-oesophageal reflux disease and dental lesions. Aliment Pharmacol Ther 2008;27: 1179–86.

62. Wan Nik WN, Banerjee A, Moazzez R. Gastro-oesophageal reflux disease symptoms and tooth wear in patients with Sjögren's syndrome. Caries Res 2011;45:323–6.

Management of Xerostomia and Other Complications of Sjögren's Syndrome

Andres Pinto, DMD, MPH, FDS RCSEd

KEYWORDS

• Sjögren's syndrome • Xerostomia • GRADE • Management • Systematic review

KEY POINTS

- Xerostomia and salivary hypofunction are the most common oral complications of Sjögren's syndrome (SS).
- Oral burning, dysphagia, and taste abnormalities are additional complaints seen in SS.
- There is low evidence on the efficacy of interventions for oral burning, dysphagia, and taste disorders in SS.
- Sialogogues have moderate to high evidence of efficacy for the management of xerostomia and salivary hypofunction in SS.

Xerostomia and salivary gland hypofunction are well-documented oral complications of SS. Xerostomia is defined as patient perception of oral dryness, whereas salivary hypofunction is the objective validation of oral dryness based on flow measurement.[1,2] The latter is a major complication of SS and is directly linked to the diagnosis of this condition.[2,3] Additional oral complications have recently been described as more is documented about the oral sequelae of this disorder. The purpose of this article is to perform a systematic review of the published literature in English, focusing on the management of the oral complications of SS (excluding dental caries). Definitions of these complications are discussed in an article by Napeñas and Rouleau in this issue.

METHODS
Search Strategy

Based on several discussions with experts in SS, the author selected the following oral complications of SS: xerostomia and salivary gland hypofunction, oral lesions, sensory complaints (oral burning, dysphagia, and dysgeusia) and fungal infections. The search strategy was defined with the help of a medical informationist and a detailed description is found in the Appendix 1. The terms used to formulate the review questions (and inclusion criteria) are presented in **Table 1**. The search was performed in PubMed (Medline), in English and included the published literature between January 1, 1950, and May 31, 2013.

The abstracts of identified articles were reviewed by the author. Relevant full-text articles were selected to be included in the final review. The selection process is described in **Fig. 1**. Bibliographies of selected articles were reviewed in detail to find additional studies that may have been missed by the initial search. Additional effort was done to contact authors of primary articles for suggestions of studies not included in the initial selection.

The authors do not report any significant financial disclosures.

Department of Oral and Maxillofacial Medicine and Diagnostic Sciences, University Hospitals Case Medical Center and Case Western Reserve University School of Dental Medicine, 2124 Cornell Road, Room 1190, Cleveland, OH 44106, USA

E-mail address: andres.pinto@uhhospitals.org

Oral Maxillofacial Surg Clin N Am 26 (2014) 63–73
http://dx.doi.org/10.1016/j.coms.2013.09.010

Table 1
Study question

Study Question	PICO Format
Population	Patients diagnosed with SS (primary or secondary)
Intervention	Clinical trials, controlled studies, controlled clinical trials, comparative studies, and meta-analysis
Control group	SS patients using comparator medication or placebo (when available)
Outcome	Subjective or objective improvement in oral dryness, number and/or frequency of oral lesions, oral burning, dysgeusia, dysphagia, clinical resolution of oral fungal infection

Data Abstraction and Evidence Grading

Study characteristics were abstracted to data forms for evidence rating. Rating was done independently for each selected complication of SS. Guidelines and free software provided by the Grading of Recommendations Assessment, Development and Evaluation (GRADE) group were followed for form development and to assess the available evidence.[4–6] Briefly, studies were assessed for risk of bias, inconsistency of the direction of results across studies, precision of effect estimates, use of surrogate outcomes (indirectness), and publication bias (available at: http://www.gradeworkinggroup.org/index.htm) **(Table 2)**.

RESULTS
Xerostomia and Salivary Hypofunction

Extensive literature has been published focusing on the effect of therapeutic interventions for the management of xerostomia and reduced salivary flow in SS: 43 studies included assessment of changes in perception of oral dryness or salivary flow[1–3,7–46]; 37 had sialometry as a primary or secondary outcome; 15 studies included randomization across groups in their study design **(Table 3)**[1,14,16,17,19,20,24,26,27,30,31,36,37,39,45]; and 5 studies included a crossover design with different washout periods.[8,9,15,17,22] Additional study designs that addressed xerostomia or hypofunction were pilot short-term trials, safety trials, placebo-controlled (not randomized) trials, and quasiexperimental observational designs. Two studies were systematic reviews of therapeutic trials for the management of dry mouth.[2,18] The Cochrane review published in 2011[18] was limited to topical therapies for xerostomia and reported low evidence to support the efficacy a specific intervention. Local salivary stimulation and moisture reservoirs showed promising results for future trials. The systematic review published in 2002[2] did not consider trials that involved cevimeline, a muscarinic agonist that was reaching the international market at that point. The same review identified 2 trials with low bias that included SS patients; both were interventions with a systemic sialagogue medication (pilocarpine).

Among the trials that randomized subjects to comparator or placebo versus intervention arm, 5 evaluated systemic sialagogues,[16,24,31,45,47] 3 evaluated local interventions (electric stimulation or moisture/lubricant reservoir),[14,17,39] and 10

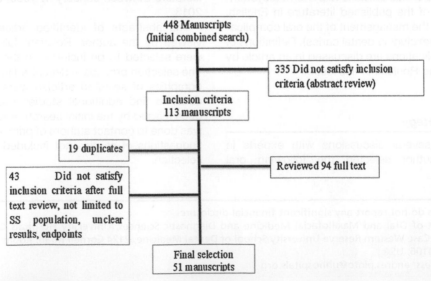

Fig. 1. Search flow diagram.

448 Manuscripts (Initial combined search)

335 Did not satisfy inclusion criteria (abstract review)

Inclusion criteria 113 manuscripts

19 duplicates

Reviewed 94 full text

43   Did not satisfy inclusion criteria after full text review, not limited to SS population, unclear results, endpoints

Final selection 51 manuscripts

Table 2
GRADE elements for evidence rating

Critical Assessment of Study Quality								
Risk of bias[a]	Inconsistency of results[a]	Indirectness[a]	Precision[a]	Publication bias[a]	Effect size[b]	Dose response[b]	Confounding (control for)[b]	Demonstrate a spurious effect[b]

Studies with the highest quality are randomized controlled trials, followed by observational studies. GRADE's suggested rating is categorical scale (high, moderate, low, and very low). Raters must incorporate the elements described in the table when rating overall quality. These are divided into factors that are considered study weaknesses[a] or strengths.[b]

  [a] Factors that downgrade the study quality.
  [b] Factors that add to the study quality.
  Data from Karanicolas PJ, Montori VM, Devereaux PJ, et al. A new "mechanistic-practical" framework for designing and interpreting randomized trials. J Clin Epidemiol 2009;62(5):479–84; and Schunemann H, Hill S, Guyatt G, et al. The GRADE approach and Bradford Hill's criteria for causation. J Epidemiol Community Health 2011;65(5):392–5.

addressed other systemic pharmacologic therapy, 5 of which evaluated the effect of systemic immune modulators on signs and symptoms of SS.[1,26,27,36,37]

Sialagogues

Fife and colleagues[16] treated 75 SS subjects with cevimeline (30 mg 3 times a day), cevimeline (60 mg 3 times a day), or placebo for 6 weeks. The 30-mg dose was significantly correlated with subjective improvement in SS status, including dry mouth. The investigators reported a withdrawal rate of 20% due to side effects of treatment. Allocation concealment was not described in enough detail, and the precision of the effect estimates was broad, possibly related to the small sample size. Leung and colleagues[24] treated 50 SS subjects (combined primary and secondary SS) over 24 weeks with cevimeline (30 mg 3 times a day) or placebo. Outcome measures included quality-of-life assessment and sialometry. Cevimeline was associated with improvement in subjective but not objective measures (flow). Period effects and carryover effects were present and may have influenced the outcome.

Petrone and colleagues[31] performed a 12-week, double-blind, randomized, placebo-controlled trial in 197 SS subjects, estimating the efficacy of cevimeline (15-mg doses 3 times a day) and cevimeline (30-mg doses 3 times a day) versus placebo. The primary efficacy endpoint was a global impression of dryness (ocular and oral) in addition to objective measures of tear and whole salivary flow. This multicenter trial had low evidence of bias and indirectness as surrogate and direct measures were implemented. Outcomes were precise, in particular, whole saliva evaluation. The randomization scheme was adequately reported, although details surrounding blinding and allocation

concealment were insufficient. Nevertheless, primary and secondary efficacy endpoints were well established and appraised with appropriate reliability. The remaining studies by Wu and colleagues[45] and Vivino and colleagues[47] were good methodologic trials assessing different doses of pilocarpine in the treatment of xerostomia and salivary hypofunction.

Local interventions

da Silva Marques and colleagues[14] compared 2 salivary stimulating interventions in a sample of 80 SS subjects. Their article was of high methodologic quality and addressed the impact of the interventions on salivary pH and volume. Frost and colleagues[17] described, in a single-blind randomized trial, the effect of an intraoral lubricating device on the oral environment of 29 SS subjects. There was no significant effect of the device on salivary flow, although it did alter the local microbiological environment. A study by Strietzel and colleagues[39] compared the use of active (electric stimulator) and inactive oral appliances in 114 subjects for 1 month. The investigators reported a significant effect on reported xerostomia with the active appliance. This effect was prolonged during a second open-label phase of the trial and included improved resting (unstimulated) salivary flow.

Immune modulators

Cummins and colleagues[1] did a randomized, parallel-group, double-blind, clinical trial of interferon versus placebo delivered oromucosally on 497 SS subjects. This trial demonstrated an effect of interferon on whole unstimulated salivary flow. The results were not positive regarding subject perception of oral dryness. The investigators hypothesized that a large placebo effect was responsible for this finding. Mariette and colleagues[26] and

Table 3
Characteristics of select randomized clinical trials on the management of xerostomia and salivary hypofunction (published in the past 5 years)

Author, Year	Design	Number of Subjects	Intervention	Results[a]	Comments
da Silva Marques et al,[14] 2011	Double-blind, randomized controlled	40 in active group 40 in comparator	Two gustatory stimulants of salivary secretion (compared): active—xylitol and fluoride, malic acid and comparator—citric acid	The active stimulant had an absolute risk reduction of 52.78% (95% CI, 33.42–72.13) in erosion potential over the comparator, fewer episodes of pH <4.5	Adequate estimation of sample size, randomization scheme. Convenience sample. WSF 0.2 mg/mL threshold to include in the study.
Strietzel et al,[39] 2011	Phase 1: randomized controlled trial of electric stimulator intraoral appliance	114 mixed xerostomia, including 66 SS	Electric intraoral stimulator vs sham appliance	Significant effect on xerostomia severity (P<.002) and frequency (P<.05) but not on flow	Possible bias with subjects on sham. 4-wk follow-up may have limited ability to detect effect. Multisite trial. No precision estimates.
Meijer et al,[27] 2010	Randomized, double blind, placebo controlled	30 SS	Rituximab or placebo infusion at days 1 and 15	Increase WSF (P = .038)	Pilot trial. WSF threshold for inclusion of >0.15 mL/min. No precision estimates.
Leung et al,[24] 2008	Randomized, double blind, placebo controlled, crossover	50 SS (22 primary SS and 28 secondary SS)	Cevimeline, 30 mg, or placebo 3 times per day	Significant improvement in xerostomia (P = .001) but not in WSF	Sample size estimation, no mention of threshold salivary flow for inclusion. Used a valid xerostomia inventory/oral QOL assessment.

Abbreviations: QOL, quality of life; WSF, whole stimulated flow.

[a] Results refer to xerostomia and salivary flow. Most studies reported additional endpoints.

Meijer and colleagues[27] investigated the efficacy of infliximab and rituximab in the treatment of SS. These trials produced conflicting results. Marriette and colleagues enrolled 103 subjects who were infused at weeks 0, 2, and 6 and followed to week 22. Multiple endpoints were assessed, including salivary flow, which did not change significantly with treatment. The study by Meijer and colleagues used rituximab (given at days 1 and 15) versus placebo on a sample of 29 SS subjects who were followed for up to 48 weeks. Significant improvement in salivary flow was evident at follow-up. Additional studies on the efficacy of etanercept by Sankar and colleagues[36] (on a sample of 29 SS subjects) and the use of low-level doxycycline to decrease SS symptoms did not report a significant effect on salivary flow.[37]

The overall rating of the evidence supporting interventions for xerostomia and salivary hypofunction in SS is moderate. The strongest evidence remains on systemic sialagogues with several accurate trials reporting efficacy of pilocarpine and cevimeline.

Oral Lesions

Despite isolated case reports of development of oral ulceration or other oral lesions in SS patients, the current search was unable to find a clinical trial that addressed the question of management of these lesions. Oral lesions have been reported in autoimmune disorders, including lupus and other rheumatologic diagnoses.[48] Some of these have an immune cause, such as lichen planus, and may occur in secondary SS, as a sign of the primary disorder. Furthermore, the association between SS and the development of oral mucosal pathology remains elusive, because many oral reactions can be triggered by topical or systemic therapy used to treat SS. The rating for the evidence is low for the management of oral lesions in SS due to lack of clinical data to support it.

Sensory Complaints

Oral burning
Six studies included oral burning as a secondary outcome measure[3,8,9,12,22,49]: 1 was a placebo-controlled trial,[49] 2 were single-blind controlled trials,[8,9] 3 were crossover trials (1 double blind),[8,9,22] and 2 were open-label trials.[3,12] Five studies compared topical/local interventions addressing xerostomia with either placebo or used subjects as their own controls. One used hydroxychloroquine as systemic therapy for SS. One study was limited to secondary SS subjects. Statistical improvement of burning sensation was reported in the placebo-controlled clinical trial.[49] This

multisite clinical trial (3 sites) tested the hypothesis that an electric stimulator could increase salivary flow in SS subjects treated over 4 weeks. A total of 77 subjects were randomly assigned to either an active arm (stimulator) or a placebo arm with a sham stimulator. The primary outcome was change in salivary flow over time, and the investigators also observed changes in other sensory complaints that included burning sensation.

The 2 single-blind trials reported conflicting results. Alpoz and colleagues[8] reported no significant change in burning in 29 subjects treated with Xialine in a crossover trial. The primary outcome in this study was the impact of the topical solution on xerostomia-related sensory complaints in this group. The results of the study highlighted patient acceptance and comfort with the study drug as a major finding, in spite of negative associations with changes in burning sensation. This study had a short follow-up time (14 days) and significant issues with precision and bias given its single-blind nature. The second single-blind trial was also one of the crossover trials; 21 SS subjects were enrolled for a 90-day trial of a commercial gel used 3 times per day. During this time they were followed twice and a new gel given (placebo) after 1 week washout for another 90 days. Strictly speaking, this trial was not a crossover because the sample was not divided into 2 groups (probably because of the sample size). Nevertheless, the follow-up was long, and the 7 subjects who had oral burning complaints had complete recovery with the use of the study medication compared with placebo. In spite of the favorable response, significant issues were the blinding of the study as well as the small sample size and lack of effect size reporting.

Cankaya and colleagues[12] reported, in an open-label trial of hydroxycloroquine in 30 SS women, no significant improvement in oral burning at 6, 12, 18, 24, and 30 week follow-up. These findings raise the possibility that the effect of topical treatment on burning complaints may be greater than the effect of systemic pharmacologic approaches and could be time dependent. The overall evaluation of the evidence on interventions for oral burning was considered low.

Dysphagia
Ten studies addressed dysphagia as a secondary outcome of interventions in SS subjects.[3,8,9,12,23,29,37,39,49,50] Five of these were described in the oral burning intervention section. Three of the 10 studies were randomized controlled clinical trials, 1 of them involving multiple sites.[23,37,39] The study by Strietzel and colleagues[39] included a total of 114 SS and mixed dry mouth subjects who were randomized to

an electric stimulator or placebo. The primary outcome was changes in resting and stimulated salivary flow, and the study was divided into 2 stages. The initial stage was a randomized controlled study where subjects were assigned to the active stimulator or placebo and followed-up for a month. This phase reported significant improvement in swallowing in the SS group (n of 66) compared with the sham appliance. This result was not maintained in the second phase of the study, a 3-month open-label trial that aimed to test long-term effects of use.

Khurshudian[23] performed a pilot randomized trial in 12 SS subjects who received 150 IU of interferon-α or placebo 3 times a day for 24 weeks. Five subjects who received interferon-α (of a total of 8 in this arm) were followed for an additional 24 weeks. Results from this group revealed improvement in swallowing function. Therefore, the swallowing positive outcome was a product of long-term use of the medication in the open-label phase.

The third randomized clinical trial was a double-blind crossover trial published by Seitsalo and colleagues.[37] This study randomized 22 SS subjects to low-dose doxycycline (20 mg) or placebo taken twice a day for 10 days. The hypothesis behind this design was that low dose of this antibiotic may have an important effect on the severity of the clinical symptoms of SS via reduction of metalloproteinase activity. Final results were not supportive of this statement for any endpoint, including swallowing capacity. The overall ranking of the evidence in this section was low. Most studies were observational and the few randomized trials were not conclusive. The study by Strietzel and colleagues offers the most evidence for short-term relief of dysphagia in SS individuals using an electric stimulator. The study was not powered, however, to assess dysphagia as a primary outcome.

Dysgeusia (taste disorders)

Negoro and colleagues[51] described a positive association between the prevalence of taste dysfunction and salivary flow in SS. In this publication, the investigators hypothesized that taste discrimination was inversely correlated to salivary flow. Their preliminary results offer an interesting hypothesis to be tested in future clinical trials. Four observational studies included taste changes as secondary outcomes.[3,8,9,52] No controlled clinical trial was identified. Two studies were single blind; 1 was double blind.[8,9,52] Two studies incorporated a crossover design with different washout periods.[8,52] All studies used convenience samples and none had a sample size calculation aimed at the taste outcome. Methodologic heterogeneity

led to broad differences in reported effects of therapy, with unclear or unreported effects in 2 studies and conflicting results from the other 2. The overall ranking of the evidence was low for management of taste disorders in SS. The absence of randomized controlled trials and shortcomings in the consistency of effect reporting in the existent observational trials deter from their contribution.

Fungal Infections

The development of oral fungal infections in SS is an expected complication of oral dryness and possible changes in salivary composition. Only 1 study was found that indirectly addressed the management of oral candidiasis in SS.[53] This open-label trial in 6 subjects with nystatin-resistant denture candidiasis tested the antifungal properties of 5% amorolfine, a medication used in dermatology to treat nail fungal infections. The varnish was applied once to twice a week on the denture and all subjects but 1 were infection-free after the final application. This subject was suspected to have SS.

The sample in this case series was composed of diverse subjects and there was no intervention to address oral fungal infection in one individual with suspected SS. Intuitively, SS poses a clinical scenario for the development of severe fungal infections. Aggressive systemic management of these infections in SS patients may seem reasonable, considering the high resistance rate to topical antifungal agents. This statement, unfortunately, is yet to be supported by well-designed clinical research. The overall ranking of the evidence on the management of oral fungal infections in SS was very low.

DISCUSSION

Evidence-based evaluation of the literature considers multiple factors that may affect study results. The most robust study design to test efficacy of interventions is the randomized, placebo-controlled, double-blind, clinical trial. Other study designs are important for hypothesis generation and pilot testing. Several well-designed clinical trials are needed to elucidate the application of an intervention to clinical practice. The important elements to evaluate in these trials are the appropriate estimation of a sample size to include in the trial, protection of blinding and allocation, randomization scheme, limitation of bias (in sample/control selection, data entry, or study process) and confounding, reporting of precise estimates with accurate effect size, and definition of clinically important difference. The latter is of major importance because it assists astute clinicians evaluate the applicability of the intervention to their patients. Many studies failed to consider the clinical importance in changes of salivary flow. Some included global estimates of change in their patient outcomes, which can easily be correlated to the numeric change in salivary flow. This is an important standardized outcome to consider in future trials. A definition of clinically importance difference in xerostomia measures has been recently proposed.[54]

The management of xerostomia and other oral signs and symptoms of SS remains a concern. The strongest evidence on effective interventions remains on the use of systemic sialagogue medications. Topical use of salivary lubricants or substitutes in severe SS has proved equivocal, and the effects of topical moisturizers seem marginal in this population. Given the broad range of severity of salivary hypofunction in SS subjects, it is yet unclear whether salivary replacement on its own is sufficient. The impact of continuous use of systemic sialagogues on different phases of SS is still unknown, and it is assumed that a minimal amount of salivary function is required for these medications to work.

The low to very low quality of interventions aimed at management of other oral signs and symptoms of SS follows the scant numbers of randomized clinical trials that address these conditions. This review was unable to find randomized clinical trials for conditions such as oral lesions or management of recurrent fungal infections in SS. Detailed protocols exist on the management of oral fungal infections in healthy subjects and other comorbidities, and SS patients are at an increased risk for development of this complication. Appropriate management may be more intensive than the published systemic or local antifugal therapy guidelines.

A novel approach to the management of rheumatologic disorders is the use of intravenous monoclonal antibodies to modulate autoimmune response. Several therapeutic agents have been evaluated in SS with equivocal results. Although few open-label trials have reported significant improvement in xerostomia and salivary flow, pilot clinical randomized trials and other larger trials have not found a significant effect. These studies have evaluated different dosing strategies and have follow-up periods ranging from 12 weeks to 48 weeks. The evidence supporting these interventions for the management of dry mouth is still to be determined.

The scoring of the evidence in SS trials is hindered by small sample sizes, lack of formal sample calculation (with few exceptions), mix of primary and secondary SS patients, and measurement of whole stimulated and unstimulated saliva in different trials. Trials should evaluate both effects on subjects' perception of dry mouth (xerostomia) and clinical salivary flow. It is also suggested that inclusion criteria specify minimal threshold levels of salivary flow and that data analysis stratifies, when possible, subgroups of baseline flow. The impact of the intervention would be clearer if these strategies were followed when planning a clinical trial.

LIMITATIONS

Some limitations exist in this systematic review. The search strategy was limited to published articles in English and the author used a single electronic database, albeit with broad coverage, for the structured search. The gray literature (ie, conference proceedings, abstracts, and unpublished dissertations) was not searched in a systematic way, and articles/studies published as meeting abstracts and in other languages may have been missed. The GRADE instrument is a robust approach to quality assessment, although it has been criticized for lacking quantitative measures. Hence, evaluation of the factors involved in the evidence ranking has to be done by individuals familiar with the critical appraisal of the scientific literature and knowledge of basic epidemiologic methods.

The availability of effect estimates, with the exception of salivary flow measures, was limited. Many authors reported statistically significant findings that did not offer precision estimates (95% CI) nor were they easily derived from the published data.

SUMMARY

The challenge when evaluating the effect of management therapies in SS is the heterogeneity in study designs and high risk of bias in a vast number of published studies to date. Few studies have robust methods and adequately report the process of study design, randomization, blinding, allocation, and outcome measures. A major identified gap was the lack of formal sample size estimates, the use of convenient sampling strategies, and the lack of blinded allocation/information about the selection of control groups. Evidence on the management of xerostomia and salivary hypofunction in SS is moderate, with most of the weight toward systemic sialagogue medication (pilocarpine and cevimeline). Although these interventions have a moderate level of evidence, their external validity to the wide SS population remains to be understood. Other interventions for recently described oral signs and symptoms of SS are still in their infancy (hypothesis generating trials) with low level of supporting evidence. Studies with systemic immune modulators successfully implemented in other rheumatologic disorders have yielded conflicting results in SS. The effect of these therapies in primary versus secondary SS is unknown.

Although the primary concern with the oral care of SS patients is their salivary flow due to the known soft tissue and dental consequences, the onset of symptoms, such as oral burning, dysphagia, and dysgeusia, should be studied further. The prevalence of these complaints may be associated with salivary hypofunction and has been previously underreported rather than a being a new occurrence.

REFERENCES

1. Cummins MJ, Papas A, Kammer GM, et al. Treatment of primary Sjogren's syndrome with low-dose human interferon alfa administered by the oromucosal route: combined phase III results. Arthritis Rheum 2003;49(4):585–93.

2. Brennan MT, Shariff G, Lockhart PB, et al. Treatment of xerostomia: a systematic review of therapeutic trials. Dent Clin North Am 2002;46(4):847–56.

3. Aliko A, Alushi A, Tafaj A, et al. Evaluation of the clinical efficacy of Biotene Oral Balance in patients with secondary Sjogren's syndrome: a pilot study. Rheumatol Int 2012;32(9):2877–81.

4. Guyatt GH, Oxman AD, Vist GE, et al. GRADE: an emerging consensus on rating quality of evidence and strength of recommendations. BMJ 2008; 336(7650):924–6.

5. Karanicolas PJ, Montori VM, Devereaux PJ, et al. A new "mechanistic-practical" framework for designing and interpreting randomized trials. J Clin Epidemiol 2009;62(5):479–84.

6. Schunemann H, Hill S, Guyatt G, et al. The GRADE approach and Bradford Hill's criteria for causation. J Epidemiol Community Health 2011;65(5):392–5.

7. Aframian DJ, Helcer M, Livni D, et al. Pilocarpine treatment in a mixed cohort of xerostomic patients. Oral Dis 2007;13(1):88–92.

8. Alpoz E, Guneri P, Onder G, et al. The efficacy of Xialine in patients with Sjogren's syndrome: a single-blind, cross-over study. Clin Oral Investig 2008;12(2):165–72.

9. Alves MB, Motta AC, Messina WC, et al. Saliva substitute in xerostomic patients with primary Sjogren's syndrome: a single-blind trial. Quintessence Int 2004;35(5):392–6.

10. Bikker A, van Woerkom JM, Kruize AA, et al. Clinical efficacy of leflunomide in primary Sjogren's

11. Blom M, Lundeberg T. Long-term follow-up of patients treated with acupuncture for xerostomia and the influence of additional treatment. Oral Dis 2000;6(1):15–24.

12. Cankaya H, Alpoz E, Karabulut G, et al. Effects of hydroxychloroquine on salivary flow rates and oral complaints of Sjogren patients: a prospective sample study. Oral Surg Oral Med Oral Pathol Oral Radiol Endod 2010;110(1):62–7.

13. Ciccia F, Giardina A, Rizzo A, et al. Rituximab modulates the expression of IL-22 in the salivary glands of patients with primary Sjogren's syndrome. Ann Rheum Dis 2013;72(5):782–3.

14. da Silva Marques DN, da Mata AD, Patto JM, et al. Effects of gustatory stimulants of salivary secretion on salivary pH and flow in patients with Sjogren's syndrome: a randomized controlled trial. J Oral Pathol Med 2011;40(10):785–92.

15. Epstein JB, Decoteau WE, Wilkinson A. Effect of Sialor in treatment of xerostomia in Sjogren's syndrome. Oral Surg Oral Med Oral Pathol 1983;56(5):495–9.

16. Fife RS, Chase WF, Dore RK, et al. Cevimeline for the treatment of xerostomia in patients with Sjogren syndrome: a randomized trial. Arch Intern Med 2002;162(11):1293–300.

17. Frost PM, Shirlaw PJ, Challacombe SJ, et al. Impact of wearing an intra-oral lubricating device on oral health in dry mouth patients. Oral Dis 2006;12(1):57–62.

18. Furness S, Worthington HV, Bryan G, et al. Interventions for the management of dry mouth: topical therapies. Cochrane Database Syst Rev 2011;(12):CD008934.

19. Gescuk B, Wu AJ, Whitcher JP, et al. Lamivudine is not effective in primary Sjogren's syndrome. Ann Rheum Dis 2005;64(9):1326–30.

20. Haila S, Koskinen A, Tenovuo J. Effects of homeopathic treatment on salivary flow rate and subjective symptoms in patients with oral dryness: a randomized trial. Homeopathy 2005;94(3):175–81.

21. Ichikawa Y, Tokunaga M, Shimizu H, et al. Clinical trial of ambroxol (Mucosolvan) in Sjogren's syndrome. Tokai J Exp Clin Med 1988;13(3):165–9.

22. Johansson G, Andersson G, Edwardsson S, et al. Effects of mouthrinses with linseed extract Salinum without/with chlorhexidine on oral conditions in patients with Sjogren's syndrome. A double-blind crossover investigation. Gerodontology 2001; 18(2):87–94.

23. Khurshudian AV. A pilot study to test the efficacy of oral administration of interferon-alpha lozenges to patients with Sjogren's syndrome. Oral Surg Oral Med Oral Pathol Oral Radiol Endod 2003;95(1):38–44.

syndrome is associated with regulation of T-cell activity and upregulation of IL-7 receptor alpha expression. Ann Rheum Dis 2012;71(12):1934–41.

24. Leung KC, McMillan AS, Wong MC, et al. The efficacy of cevimeline hydrochloride in the treatment of xerostomia in Sjogren's syndrome in southern Chinese patients: a randomised double-blind, placebo-controlled crossover study. Clin Rheumatol 2008;27(4):429–36.

25. Malmstrom MJ, Segerberg-Konttinen M, Tuominen TS, et al. Xerostomia due to Sjogren's syndrome. Diagnostic criteria, treatment and outlines for a continuous dental care programme and an open trial with Sulfarlem. Scand J Rheumatol 1988;17(2):77–86.

26. Mariette X, Ravaud P, Steinfeld S, et al. Inefficacy of infliximab in primary Sjogren's syndrome: results of the randomized, controlled Trial of Remicade in Primary Sjogren's Syndrome (TRIPSS). Arthritis Rheum 2004;50(4):1270–6.

27. Meijer JM, Meiners PM, Vissink A, et al. Effectiveness of rituximab treatment in primary Sjogren's syndrome: a randomized, double-blind, placebo-controlled trial. Arthritis Rheum 2010;62(4):960–8.

28. Miyawaki S, Nishiyama S, Matoba K. Efficacy of low-dose prednisolone maintenance for saliva production and serological abnormalities in patients with primary Sjogren's syndrome. Intern Med 1999;38(12):938–43.

29. Nakayamada S, Saito K, Umehara H, et al. Efficacy and safety of mizoribine for the treatment of Sjogren's syndrome: a multicenter open-label clinical trial. Mod Rheumatol 2007;17(6):464–9.

30. Pedersen A, Gerner N, Palmvang I, et al. LongoVital in the treatment of Sjogren's syndrome. Clin Exp Rheumatol 1999;17(5):533–8.

31. Petrone D, Condemi JJ, Fife R, et al. A double-blind, randomized, placebo-controlled study of cevimeline in Sjogren's syndrome patients with xerostomia and keratoconjunctivitis sicca. Arthritis Rheum 2002;46(3):748–54.

32. Pijpe J, Meijer JM, Bootsma H, et al. Clinical and histologic evidence of salivary gland restoration supports the efficacy of rituximab treatment in Sjogren's syndrome. Arthritis Rheum 2009;60(11):3251–6.

33. Pijpe J, van Imhoff GW, Spijkervet FK, et al. Rituximab treatment in patients with primary Sjogren's syndrome: an open-label phase II study. Arthritis Rheum 2005;52(9):2740–50.

34. Rhodus NL, Schuh MJ. Effects of pilocarpine on salivary flow in patients with Sjogren's syndrome. Oral Surg Oral Med Oral Pathol 1991;72(5):545–9.

35. Rihl M, Ulbricht K, Schmidt RE, et al. Treatment of sicca symptoms with hydroxychloroquine in patients with Sjogren's syndrome. Rheumatology (Oxford) 2009;48(7):796–9.

36. Sankar V, Brennan MT, Kok MR, et al. Etanercept in Sjogren's syndrome: a twelve-week randomized, double-blind, placebo-controlled pilot clinical trial. Arthritis Rheum 2004;50(7):2240–5.

37. Seitsalo H, Niemela RK, Marinescu-Gava M, et al. Effectiveness of low-dose doxycycline (LDD) on clinical symptoms of Sjogren's syndrome: a randomized, double-blind, placebo controlled crossover study. J Negat Results Biomed 2007;6:11.

38. Steinfeld SD, Tant L, Burmester GR, et al. Epratuzumab (humanised anti-CD22 antibody) in primary Sjogren's syndrome: an open-label phase I/II study. Arthritis Res Ther 2006;8(4):R129.

39. Strietzel FP, Lafaurie GI, Mendoza GR, et al. Efficacy and safety of an intraoral electrostimulation device for xerostomia relief: a multicenter, randomized trial. Arthritis Rheum 2011;63(1):180–90.

40. Sugai S, Takahashi H, Ohta S, et al. Efficacy and safety of rebamipide for the treatment of dry mouth symptoms in patients with Sjogren's syndrome: a double-blind placebo controlled multicenter trial. Mod Rheumatol 2009;19(2):114–24.

41. Takagi Y, Katayama I, Tashiro S, et al. Parotid irrigation and cevimeline gargle for treatment of xerostomia in Sjogren's syndrome. J Rheumatol 2008; 35(11):2289–91.

42. ter Borg EJ, Haanen HC, Haas FJ, et al. Treatment of primary Sjogren's syndrome with D-penicillamine: a pilot study. Neth J Med 2002;60(10):402–6.

43. van Woerkom JM, Kruize AA, Geenen R, et al. Safety and efficacy of leflunomide in primary Sjogren's syndrome: a phase II pilot study. Ann Rheum Dis 2007;66(8):1026–32.

44. Willeke P, Schluter B, Becker H, et al. Mycophenolate sodium treatment in patients with primary Sjogren syndrome: a pilot trial. Arthritis Res Ther 2007; 9(6):R115.

45. Wu CH, Hsieh SC, Lee KL, et al. Pilocarpine hydrochloride for the treatment of xerostomia in patients with Sjogren's syndrome in Taiwan–a double-blind, placebo-controlled trial. J Formos Med Assoc 2006;105(10):796–803.

46. Zandbelt MM, de Wilde P, van Damme P, et al. Etanercept in the treatment of patients with primary Sjogren's syndrome: a pilot study. J Rheumatol 2004;31(1):96–101.

47. Vivino FB, Al-Hashimi I, Khan Z, et al. Pilocarpine tablets for the treatment of dry mouth and dry eye symptoms in patients with Sjogren syndrome: a randomized, placebo-controlled, fixed-dose, multicenter trial. P92-01 Study Group. Arch Intern Med 1999;159(2):174–81.

48. Mays JW, Sarmadi M, Moutsopoulos NM. Oral manifestations of systemic autoimmune and inflammatory diseases: diagnosis and clinical management. J Evid Based Dent Pract 2012; 12(Suppl 3):265–82.

49. Talal N, Quinn JH, Daniels TE. The clinical effects of electrostimulation on salivary function of Sjogren's syndrome patients. A placebo controlled study. Rheumatol Int 1992;12(2):43–5.

50. Kasama T, Shiozawa F, Isozaki T, et al. Effect of the H2 receptor antagonist nizatidine on xerostomia in patients with primary Sjogren's syndrome. Mod Rheumatol 2008;18(5):455–9.

51. Negoro A, Umemoto M, Fujii M, et al. Taste function in Sjogren's syndrome patients with special reference to clinical tests. Auris Nasus Larynx 2004; 31(2):141–7.

52. Gravenmade EJ, Vissink A. Mucin-containing lozenges in the treatment of intraoral problems associated with Sjogren's syndrome. A double-blind crossover study in 42 patients. Oral Surg Oral Med Oral Pathol 1993;75(4): 466–71.

53. Milillo L, Lo Muzio L, Carlino P, et al. Candida-related denture stomatitis: a pilot study of the efficacy of an amorolfine antifungal varnish. Int J Prosthodont 2005;18(1):55–9.

54. Thomson WM. Measuring change in dry-mouth symptoms over time using the Xerostomia Inventory. Gerodontology 2007;24(1):30–5.

APPENDIX 1: SEARCH STRATEGY

Search strategies: PubMed
Jan 1, 1950 - May 31, 2013

Study type: comparative study, clinical trial, controlled clinical trial, randomized controlled trial, meta-analysis.

XEROSTOMIA AND SJOGREN SYNDROME
Salivary Hypofunction AND Sjogren Syndrome

Treatment OR therapy

(("organization and administration"[MeSH Terms] OR ("organization"[All Fields] AND "administration"[All Fields]) OR "organization and administration"[All Fields] OR "management"[All Fields] OR "disease management"[MeSH Terms] OR ("disease"[All Fields] AND "management"[All Fields]) OR "disease management"[All Fields]) AND ("xerostomia"[MeSH Terms] OR "xerostomia"[All Fields])) AND ("sjogren's syndrome"[MeSH Terms] OR ("sjogren's"[All Fields] AND "syndrome"[All Fields]) OR "sjogren's syndrome"[All Fields] OR ("sjogren"[All Fields] AND "syndrome"[All Fields]) OR "sjogren syndrome"[All Fields]) AND (Clinical Trial[ptyp] OR Comparative Study[ptyp] OR Controlled Clinical Trial[ptyp] OR Meta-Analysis[ptyp] OR Randomized Controlled Trial[ptyp])

(("therapy"[Subheading] OR "therapy"[All Fields] OR "treatment"[All Fields] OR "therapeutics"[MeSH Terms] OR "therapeutics"[All Fields]) AND ("xerostomia"[MeSH Terms] OR "xerostomia"[All Fields])) AND ("sjogren's syndrome"[MeSH Terms] OR ("sjogren's"[All Fields] AND "syndrome"[All Fields]) OR "sjogren's syndrome"[All Fields] OR ("sjogren"[All Fields] AND "syndrome"[All Fields])

OR "sjogren syndrome"[All Fields]) AND (Clinical Trial[ptyp] OR Comparative Study[ptyp] OR Controlled Clinical Trial[ptyp] OR Meta-Analysis [ptyp] OR Randomized Controlled Trial[ptyp])

ORAL LESIONS AND SJOGREN SYNDROME

(("mouth"[MeSH Terms] OR "mouth"[All Fields] OR "oral"[All Fields]) AND lesions[All Fields]) AND ("sjogren's syndrome"[MeSH Terms] OR ("sjogren's"[All Fields] AND "syndrome"[All Fields]) OR "sjogren's syndrome"[All Fields] OR ("sjogren"[All Fields] AND "syndrome"[All Fields]) OR "sjogren syndrome"[All Fields]) AND (Clinical Trial[ptyp] OR Comparative Study[ptyp] OR Controlled Clinical Trial[ptyp] OR Meta-Analysis[ptyp] OR Randomized Controlled Trial[ptyp])

ORAL ULCERS AND SJOGREN SYNDROME

("oral ulcer"[MeSH Terms] OR ("oral"[All Fields] AND "ulcer"[All Fields]) OR "oral ulcer"[All Fields] OR ("oral"[All Fields] AND "ulcers"[All Fields]) OR "oral ulcers"[All Fields]) AND ("sjogren's syndrome"[MeSH Terms] OR ("sjogren's"[All Fields] AND "syndrome"[All Fields]) OR "sjogren's syndrome"[All Fields] OR ("sjogren"[All Fields] AND "syndrome"[All Fields]) OR "sjogren syndrome"[All Fields]) AND (Clinical Trial[ptyp] OR Comparative Study[ptyp] OR Controlled Clinical Trial[ptyp] OR Guideline[ptyp] OR Meta-Analysis[ptyp] OR Randomized Controlled Trial[ptyp] OR systematic[sb])

Tried mouth ulcers, mouth lesions, leukoplakia, erythroplakia.

ORAL BURNING AND SJOGREN SYNDROME
Treatment OR Therapy

(("mouth"[MeSH Terms] OR "mouth"[All Fields] OR "oral"[All Fields]) AND burning[All Fields]) AND ("sjogren's syndrome"[MeSH Terms] OR ("sjogren's"[All Fields] AND "syndrome"[All Fields]) OR "sjogren's syndrome"[All Fields] OR ("sjogren"[All Fields] AND "syndrome"[All Fields]) OR "sjogren syndrome"[All Fields]) AND (Clinical Trial[ptyp] OR Comparative Study[ptyp] OR Controlled Clinical Trial[ptyp] OR Guideline[ptyp] OR Meta-Analysis[ptyp] OR Randomized Controlled Trial[ptyp] OR systematic[sb])

DYSPHAGIA AND SJOGREN SYNDROME
Treatment OR Therapy

("deglutition disorders"[MeSH Terms] OR ("deglutition"[All Fields] AND "disorders"[All Fields]) OR "deglutition disorders"[All Fields] OR "dysphagia"[All Fields]) AND ("sjogren's syndrome"[MeSH Terms] OR ("sjogren's"[All Fields] AND "syndrome"[All Fields]) OR "sjogren's syndrome"[All Fields] OR ("sjogren"[All Fields] AND "syndrome"[All Fields]) OR "sjogren syndrome"[All Fields]) AND (Clinical Trial[ptyp] OR Comparative Study[ptyp] OR Controlled Clinical Trial[ptyp] OR Guideline[ptyp] OR Meta-Analysis[ptyp] OR Randomized Controlled Trial[ptyp] OR systematic[sb])

SWALLOWING AND SJOGREN SYNDROME

("deglutition"[MeSH Terms] OR "deglutition"[All Fields] OR "swallowing"[All Fields]) AND ("sjogren's syndrome"[MeSH Terms] OR ("sjogren's"[All Fields] AND "syndrome"[All Fields]) OR "sjogren's syndrome"[All Fields] OR ("sjogren"[All Fields] AND "syndrome"[All Fields]) OR "sjogren syndrome"[All Fields]) AND Clinical Trial[ptyp]

("therapy"[Subheading] OR "therapy"[All Fields] OR "therapeutics"[MeSH Terms] OR "therapeutics"[All Fields]) AND ("deglutition"[MeSH Terms] OR "deglutition"[All Fields] OR "swallowing"[All Fields]) AND ("sjogren's syndrome"[MeSH Terms] OR ("sjogren's"[All Fields] AND "syndrome"[All Fields]) OR "sjogren's syndrome"[All Fields] OR ("sjogren"[All Fields] AND "syndrome"[All Fields]) OR "sjogren syndrome"[All Fields]) AND Clinical Trial[ptyp]

DYSGUESIA AND SJOGREN SYNDROME
Taste AND Sjogren Syndrome

Treatment OR therapy
dysgeusia[All Fields] AND sjogren syndrome[All Fields] AND ((Clinical Trial[ptyp] OR Comparative Study[ptyp] OR Controlled Clinical Trial[ptyp] OR Guideline[ptyp] OR Meta-Analysis[ptyp] OR Randomized Controlled Trial[ptyp] OR systematic[sb]))

("taste"[MeSH Terms] OR "taste"[All Fields]) AND ("sjogren's syndrome"[MeSH Terms] OR ("sjogren's"[All Fields] AND "syndrome"[All Fields]) OR "sjogren's syndrome"[All Fields] OR ("sjogren"[All Fields] AND "syndrome"[All Fields]) OR "sjogren syndrome"[All Fields]) AND (Clinical Trial[ptyp] OR Comparative Study[ptyp] OR Controlled Clinical Trial

ORAL FUNGAL INFECTION AND SJOGREN SYNDROME
Oral Candidiasis AND Sjogren Syndrome

Treatment of therapy
(("mouth"[MeSH Terms] OR "mouth"[All Fields] OR "oral"[All Fields]) AND ("mycoses"[MeSH Terms] OR "mycoses"[All Fields] OR ("fungal"[All Fields] AND "infection"[All Fields]) OR "fungal infection"[All Fields])) AND Sjogren[All Fields] AND Clinical Trial[ptyp]

("therapy"[Subheading] OR "therapy"[All Fields] OR "treatment"[All Fields] OR "therapeutics"[MeSH Terms] OR "therapeutics"[All Fields]) AND (("mouth"[MeSH Terms] OR "mouth"[All Fields] OR "oral"[All Fields]) AND ("mycoses"[MeSH Terms] OR "mycoses"[All Fields] OR ("fungal"[All Fields] AND "infection"[All Fields]) OR "fungal infection"[All Fields])) AND ("sjogren's syndrome"[MeSH Terms] OR ("sjogren's"[All Fields] AND "syndrome"[All Fields]) OR "sjogren's syndrome"[All Fields] OR ("sjogren"[All Fields] AND "syndrome"[All Fields]) OR "sjogren syndrome"[All Fields]) AND Clinical Trial[ptyp] syndrome"[All Fields] OR ("sjögren's syndrome" OR ("sjögren"[All Fields] AND "syndrome"[All Fields]) "sjögren syndrome"[All Fields] OR "sjögren syndrome"[All Fields]) AND (Clinical Trial[ptyp] OR Comparative Study[ptyp] OR Controlled Clinical Trial[ptyp] OR Guideline[ptyp] OR Meta-Analysis[ptyp] OR Randomized Controlled Trial[ptyp] OR systematic[sb])

SWALLOWING AND SJÖGREN SYNDROME

("deglutition"[MeSH Terms] OR "deglutition"[All Fields]) OR "swallowing"[All Fields] AND ("sjögren's syndrome"[MeSH Terms] OR ("sjögren's"[All Fields]) OR "sjögren's syndrome"[All Fields] OR ("sjögren's"[All Fields]) OR ("sjögren"[All Fields] AND "syndrome"[All Fields]) OR "sjögren syndrome"[All Fields]) AND Clinical Trial[ptyp])

"therapy"[Subheading] OR "therapy"[All Fields] OR "therapeutics"[MeSH Terms] OR "therapeutics"[All Fields]) AND ("deglutition"[MeSH Terms] OR "deglutition"[All Fields] OR "swallowing"[All Fields] AND ("sjögren's syndrome"[MeSH Terms] OR "sjögren's"[All Fields]) OR "syndrome"[All Fields]) OR "sjögren's syndrome"[All Fields] OR ("sjögren"[All Fields] AND "syndrome"[All Fields]) OR "sjögren syndrome"[All Fields]) AND Clinical Trial[ptyp])

DYSGEUSIA AND SJÖGREN SYNDROME
Taste AND Sjögren Syndrome

Treatment OR therapy

dysgeusia[All Fields] AND sjögren syndrome[All Fields] AND (Clinical Trial[ptyp] OR Comparative Study[ptyp] OR Controlled Clinical Trial[ptyp] OR

(Guideline[ptyp] OR Meta-Analysis[ptyp] OR Randomized Controlled Trial[ptyp] OR systematic[sb]) ("taste"[MeSH Terms] OR "taste"[All Fields] AND "sjögren's syndrome"[MeSH Terms] OR "sjögren's"[All Fields] AND "syndrome"[All Fields] OR "sjögren's syndrome"[All Fields] OR "sjögren's syndrome"[All Fields] OR "sjögren syndrome"[All Fields]) AND (Clinical Trial [ptyp] OR Comparative Study[ptyp] OR Controlled Clinical Trial

ORAL FUNGAL INFECTION AND SJÖGREN SYNDROME
Oral Candidiasis AND Sjögren Syndrome

Treatment of therapy

("mouth"[MeSH Terms] OR "mouth"[All Fields] OR "oral"[All Fields] AND ("mycoses"[MeSH Terms] OR "mycoses"[All Fields] OR ("fungal"[All Fields] AND "infection"[All Fields] OR "fungal infection" [All Fields] AND Sjögren[All Fields] AND Clinical Trial[ptyp]

("therapy"[Subheading] OR "therapy"[All Fields] OR "treatment"[All Fields] OR "therapeutics" [MeSH Terms] OR "therapeutics"[All Fields] AND ("mouth"[MeSH Terms] OR "mouth"[All Fields] OR "oral"[All Fields] AND ("mycoses"[MeSH Terms] OR "mycoses"[All Fields] OR ("fungal"[All Fields] AND "infection"[All Fields] OR "fungal infection"[MeSH Terms] AND ("sjögren's syndrome"[All Fields] OR ("sjögren's"[All Fields] OR ("sjögren's"[All Fields]) AND "syndrome"[All Fields] OR "sjögren's syndrome"[All Fields] OR "sjögren syndrome"[All Fields]) AND Clinical Trial[ptyp])

Salivary Gland Disease in Sjögren's Syndrome
Sialoadenitis to Lymphoma

Michael D. Turner, DDS, MD[a,b,*]

KEYWORDS

- Sjögren's syndrome • Lymphoma • Sialoadenitis • Autoimmune diseases • Sialoendoscopy

KEY POINTS

- Although associated genes in patients with primary Sjögren's syndrome have been identified, the clinical correlation has yet to be determined.
- There are multiple theories of what causes salivary gland dysfunction in Sjögren's syndrome, but none of them has been definitively proved.
- When acinar cells stop producing serous saliva, mucous plugs can form within the salivary glands, causing obstructive sialoadenitis, possibly leading to a salivary gland infection.
- Patients with Sjögren's syndrome can develop non-Hodgkin lymphoma, particularly mucosa-associated lymphoid tissue lymphoma. These lymphomas in turn can develop into more aggressive lymphomas.
- Lymphoma is the leading cause of death of patients with Sjögren's syndrome.

INTRODUCTION

Sjögren's syndrome (SS) is an insidious, autoimmune disease that affects both men and women. Its clinical effects, as it progresses, affect the oral, ocular, and other extraglandular exocrine systems, and it generally has a negative effect on the quality of life of patients. When the syndrome presents by itself, it is termed primary SS (pSS), and when it presents concurrently with other autoimmune disease(s), it is termed secondary SS (sSS).

The full cause of the disease is still unknown, but basic, translational, and clinical scientists, over the last 2 decades, have begun to determine genetic and cellular pathways, piecing together various clues as to why the disease occurs, how it progresses, and most importantly, why it can transform into lymphoma, which is the leading cause of death in patients with SS.

Approximately 1 million people have been diagnosed with SS in the United States, with a global estimate of 0.9% to 1.4% of the population.[1] Because of its multitude of symptoms, it is likely that there are cases that remain undiagnosed, and so the reported incidence and prevalence are most likely inaccurate.[2] Most of the patients who develop SS are women, and although it can occur at any age, it is generally seen between the ages of 40 and 60 years. For further discussion on the epidemiology of SS, please see the article by Reksten TR and Jonsson MV elsewhere in this issue.

Because of the subtle onset of the symptoms, there is an average time of 10 years between the relative onset and the confirmed diagnosis of the disease.[3] A known confounder in the recognition of SS is that the symptoms do not always present concurrently, so each symptom is treated separately, sometimes by different health care providers, causing a delay in SS identification.

a New York Center for Salivary Gland Diseases, Head and Neck Institute, Beth Israel Medical Center, New York, NY 10003, USA; b Oral and Maxillofacial Surgery, Jacobi Medical Center, Bronx, NY 10461, USA
* New York Center for Salivary Gland Diseases, Head and Neck Institute, Beth Israel Medical Center, 10 Union Square East, Suite 5B, New York, NY 10003.
E-mail address: mturner@chpnet.org

Oral Maxillofacial Surg Clin N Am 26 (2014) 75–81
http://dx.doi.org/10.1016/j.coms.2013.09.006
1042-3699/14/$ – see front matter © 2014 Elsevier Inc. All rights reserved.

The cause of the disease is still unknown, but parts of the puzzle have been identified, namely genetic predisposition and aberrant cellular function.

GENETIC PREDISPOSITION

Because of the confounding variables associated with the concurrent autoimmune diseases in sSS, genetic comparisons have focused on studies of patients with pSS and pSS specimens. In evaluating pSS specimens, it is clear that the most commonly found histocompatibility complex in pSS is on the HLA genes DR and DQ.[4] It seems that different HLA associations have been identified based on ethnicity, although currently, a focused study of these differences is difficult because of the low number of available specimens. To try to eliminate these ethnically variable genes, a meta-analysis was performed and its conclusion was published in 2012.[4] It evaluated the data from 1166 cases and 6470 controls from 23 articles from a variety of ethnicities. It was found that at the allelic level, DRB1*03:01, DQA1*05:01, DQB1*02:01, DRB1*03-DQB1*02 and DRB1*03, were found to be risk factors for pSS, and DQA1*02:01, DQA1*03:01 and DQB1*05:01 alleles were noted to be protective factors against the disease. The serologic groups DR2, DR3, DR8, DR16, DR17, DR52, DQ2 and DQ4 were also found to impart risk for developing pSS, whereas DR1 and DR7 were found to be protective in nature.

The meaning of these results is not yet clear, but it has been hypothesized that the genes create an altered peptide conformation in the HLA molecules, which makes them susceptible to autoantibody binding.[5,6] The HLA DRB1*03:01 risk allele, in an epitope binding prediction, was found to have good binding potential to the 24 peptides found in the Ro, La, and muscarinic type 3 acetylcholine (Ach) receptors (M3R) antigen molecules, 3 molecules that have been definitively linked to SS.[4]

ABERRANT CELLULAR FUNCTION

The pathophysiology of SS was first believed to be an immune-directed, autoantibody destruction of the saliva-secreting acinar cells.[7] As the ability to acquire sensitive genetic and molecular information has advanced, this simplistic model has been discounted. Regardless, the sequence of events that leads to salivary dysfunction is still not clear, but it is known that the disease progression is more complex than it was first believed to be.

The main finding in SS autoimmune pathophysiology is the interaction and aberrant function of both the cellular and humoral immune systems. The cells predominantly associated with SS are CD4 helper T Cells (Th1), B cells, and plasma cells. Although the interaction between the 2 systems in SS is not clear, 2 effects have been identified: inflammation and cellular infiltration. The combination and interaction of these 2 effects on the salivary gland cells result in the various systemic diseases associated with SS.

To understand the abnormal salivary function in SS, it is best to review the basic mechanism of salivary gland cell secretion. ACh binds to and activates the G protein-coupled M3R.[8,9] The activated G protein stimulates phospholipase C to generate inositol 1,4,5-trisphosphate (IP3), which binds to IP3 receptors on intracellular endoplasmic reticulum, which stores the intracellular calcium (Ca^{2+}). Stimulation of the IP3 receptors causes a Ca^{2+} release, and this causes a cascade that further stimulates an even larger Ca^{2+} release, which both amplifies and propagates the Ca^{2+} signal. The increase in intracellular Ca^{2+} activates apical membrane chloride (Cl^-) channels.[10] Sodium ions (Na^+) follow Cl^- across the cell to maintain electrochemical neutrality, creating an osmotic gradient across the acinar cells, and this is what draws water (the main component of saliva) into the lumen.

As with many facets of SS, the initial event is still unknown. A popular hypothesis is that the disease cascade is initiated by a virus. The virus causes a reaction in the dendritic cell (DC) and salivary gland epithelial cells, which results in the formation of certain antigens, particularly Ro, La, and M3R, which are presented to MHC-2 molecules, triggering the secretion of cytokines and chemokines, particularly interferon γ (IFN-γ). The predominance of IFN-γ–dominated Th1 in SS is now an accepted fact. Recent studies also implicate a DC subset called plasmacytoid DC, which in SS specimens produces excess interferon α (IFN-α).[11] Many other cytokines and chemokines have also been identified in varying degrees, but description of these and their effects and interactions is beyond the scope of this article.

IFN induces the expression in many (hundreds) of inflammatory and antiviral genes, particularly B-cell activating factor (BAFF) and some forms of anti-Ro (see later discussion for clinical correlation).[12]

The activation of BAFF and other cytokines causes a migration and infiltration of T and B lymphocytes into the salivary gland cells. As these lymphocytes increase in number, they are further activated by the antigens found on the gland epithelium and DCs, creating an autoimmune reaction. B cells start to produce anti-Ro and anti-La antibodies, also termed SS-A and SS-B antibodies. These 2 antibodies have been found to be important in the diagnosis of SS (see article elsewhere in this issue). Another antibody, which has been hypothesized to be present, is anti-(M3R), which could be the antibody that inactivates the salivary acinar cells and creates the gland dysfunction.

The M3R inactivation proposal is a viable hypothesis. The salivary glands of many patients with SS have large amounts of normal appearing, nonfibrosed acinar tissue, which is unable to function, as shown by the lack of salivary flow when stimulated.[13,14]

Salivary acinar tissue isolated from patients with SS is functional in vitro, although with a reduced sensitivity to threshold levels of muscarinic stimulation.[14,15] Other studies have shown that glandular atrophy is the long-term consequence of diminished function and that, in the elderly, it is possible to lose significant amounts of glandular tissue without affecting salivary flow.[16,17] Overall, these findings strongly suggest that the lack of glandular function in many patients with SS is the result of a blockage of acinar function, which is then followed by atrophy or apoptosis.[18,19] Other reports detail autonomic symptoms in patients with SS, further supporting this theory. These symptoms include bladder irritability,[20,21] Adie tonic pupil,[22] impaired microvasculature responses to cholinergic stimulation,[23] and variable heart rate.[24] All these symptoms, as well as those of xerostomia and xerophthalmia, create an inference that the blockade of M3R by antibodies is the key to the dysfunction present in the disease.[25] This hypothesis has been difficult to prove, because of the inability to isolate the M3R antibody.

CLINICAL PROGRESSION

Diagnosing SS can be difficult, so being able to identify the specific onset is confounded by the complexity of the clinical symptoms, as well as the possibility of concurrent symptoms from other autoimmune disease in sSS.

The suspicion of SS generally occurs when a patient presents with complaints of xerostomia or dry eyes. In a 2001 study, 93.5% of patients with SS had dry mouth and 13.6% had dry eyes.[26] Once the major salivary glands, particularly the parotid glands, decrease in function, a measurable decrease in unstimulated whole saliva volumes (15 mL or less) becomes evident. Similarly, the symptoms of dry eyes occurs even though lacrimal secretions are present.[27] The terms hyposalivation

and xerostomia continue to be used interchangeably and therefore create some confusion in review of the data. Xerostomia, the subjective feeling of dry mouth, does not always correlate with clinical hyposalivation, the objective findings of a decrease in saliva production. The full diagnostic criteria are discussed in the article elsewhere in this issue.

Within the mouth, the decrease in saliva has the following effects. A loss of pH buffering and mechanical cleansing causes an increase in the rate of dental caries. Chronic periodontal disease increases because of a decrease in the immune function of the saliva. The moisturizing effect of saliva results in oral mucosa inflammation and friability. Oral *Candida* infections also occur for the same reason. Ocular dryness leads to susceptibility to superficial infections, corneal abrasions, and retained foreign bodies. Please see the article elsewhere in this issue for management of xerostomia.

ENLARGEMENT OF THE PAROTID GLANDS AND SIALOADENITIS

Bilateral parotid gland enlargement has been found in 25% to 60% of all patients. The enlargement of the parotid glands can be acute or chronic. Acute bilateral or unilateral swelling associated with pain can be caused by obstruction of the salivary glands by mucous plugging, which form when the mucous secreting cells become the dominant source of the saliva (**Fig. 1**). This situation can result in a salivary gland infection by retrograde contamination from the oral cavity. The obstruction is managed by disruption of the plug. These plugs are found diffusely within the glands in the primary, secondary, and tertiary glandular ductules. Disruption of the plugs can be difficult purely using mechanical probes, because they cannot be accurately placed into the small branches of the ductules. In the last decade, these mucous plugs, like in other branching ductule systems, have been managed using endoscopy of the salivary glands, termed sialoendoscopy.[28] Sialoendoscopy allows for visualized disruption of the mucous plugs using hydrodissection and microinstrumentation. When a concurrent bacterial infection does occur, this can be managed by a multitude of antibiotics. The antibiotics must cover oral flora, typically the gram-positive cocci (eg, *Staphylococcus, Streptococcus*).[29]

Another cause of swelling is secondary to inflammation, which can be unilateral or bilateral and can be present in the parotid or the submandibular glands. When evaluated histologically, a significant infiltration of the acinar cells is present.

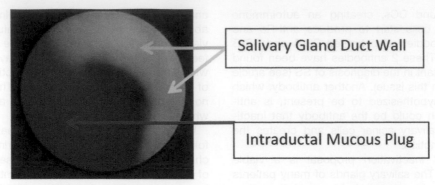

Fig. 1. Mucous plug in SS parotid gland ductule, visualized through 0.8-mm sialoendoscope.

The infiltration comprises both T cells and B cells. These lymphocytes secrete cytokines and chemokines, particularly the tumor necrosis factor α and interleukin 1α (IL-1α), as well as IL-7, IL-12, and IL-15, IFN-γ, and IL-4, causing a severe inflammatory effect.

As stated earlier, these cytokines cause further cellular chemotaxis, which then exacerbates the glandular inflammation.[30] Theories have been put forward that this infiltration replaces the salivary acinar cells, resulting in cytotoxic death and cellular apoptosis, causing the decrease and then loss of saliva production. This theory has been challenged because of the finding that there are patients with SS with no salivary flow who have noninfiltrated salivary acinar cells, lending more credence to anti-M3R deactivation of the cells (see section on aberrant cellular function).[31]

A purely inflammatory swelling can be managed by nonsteroidal antiinflammatory drugs and conservative therapy, although corticoid steroids and other antiinflammatory medications can be used to decrease the severity of the reaction. On examination, these glands are generally tender to palpation, but no pus is expressed.

LYMPHOMA

Of great concern in patients with SS is the possibility of the development of non-Hodgkin lymphoma (NHL). Studies have found, on average, that 4.3% of patients with SS develop NHL around 7.5 years (5–10 years) after initial SS diagnosis.[32] The most common lymphoma associated with SS is mucosa-associated lymphoid tissue lymphoma (MALT), a B-cell lymphoma. Although the body of evidence is still lacking, prolonged B-cell survival and excessive B-cell activity most likely result in an increased production of BAFF, increasing the risk of lymphoma formation.[33] Analysis of immunoglobulin variable regions in patients with SS and lymphoma has

found that the associated B cells produce rheumatoid factor (RF).[34,35] This constant stimulation of these RF-secreting B cells has been theorized to be the first event of lymphomagenesis in SS, although the sequence, like many pathways in SS, is unknown.[36]

The other NHL found in patients with SS is the more aggressive diffuse large B-cell lymphoma (DLBCL). Some studies have found that 10% of all SS-MALT lymphomas transform into DLBCL. The susceptibility and the theories of transformation are beyond the scope of this article.[37,38]

Clinical risk factors for the suspicion of NHL lymphoma in patients with SS are unilateral or bilateral enlargement of parotid glands, palpable purpura, splenomegaly, and lymphadenopathy and leg ulcers secondary to vasculitis, mixed cryoglobulinemia, and low C4 level.

If there is a suspicion of lymphoma from clinical signs, the most important next step is performance of a tissue biopsy. Although fine-needle and core biopsies can be performed, to diagnose the specific type of NHL, the histologic cellular architecture must be evaluated. There are also other examinations that need to be performed for staging purposes (**Box 1**).[39]

A therapeutic algorithm based on the current literature has been proposed by Routsias. Prognostic factors in a non-SS algorithm is based on the criteria of the International Prognostic Index (IPI) score (**Boxes 2 and 3**).[40] These criteria are age, stage, number of extranodal sites, performance status, and lactate dehydrogenase levels.[41]

Patients with diagnosed MALT lymphoma, but who are negative for symptoms, bone marrow infiltration, and lymphadenopathy, and have a low IPI score (0–1), are generally managed with close observation and no therapeutic treatment. This treatment has a 5-year survival rate of 90%.

Patients who have MALT lymphoma with high IPI scores and multiple nodal involvement are

<table>
<tr><td>

Box 1
NHL evaluation in patients with SS

- Incisional biopsy of extranodal tissue
- Excisional lymph node biopsies
- Evaluation of Waldeyer ring
- CT of neck, chest, abdomen, and pelvis
- Complete blood count
- Chemistry panel
- Mixed monoclonal cryoglobulinemia
- Lactate dehydrogenase level
- Serum protein electrophoresis
- Bone marrow aspiration to rule out marrow involvement
- Gastroduodenal endoscopy with biopsies
- Any pulmonary ascites should be drawn for a histologic assessment to rule out a bronchial involvement

</td></tr>
</table>

managed with rituximab alone, or in conjunction with other commonly used chemotherapeutic agents, 2-chlorodeoxyadenosine, fludarabine, and chlorambucil-cyclophosphamide, which has increased the 3-year survival rate to 80% and the disease-free rate to 80%.[39] Rituximab is a monoclonal antibody that targets the CD20 protein found on B cells. It destroys the B cells, so it is useful in the treatment of B-cell–associated diseases, particularly B-cell lymphomas.

In patients whose MALT is transforming or has transformed into DLBCL, the current therapy is CHOP (cyclophosphamide, doxorubicin, vincristine, and prednisone) with rituximab. This therapy has increased the 3-year survival rate from 37% to 100%, although these results should be considered preliminary.[42]

<table>
<tr><td>

Box 2
International Prognostic Indicator Score (IPI).
One point is assigned for each risk factor

- Age greater than 60 years
- Stage III or IV disease
- Increased serum lactate dehydrogenase level
- Eastern Cooperative Oncology Group/Zubrod performance status of 2, 3, or 4
- More than 1 extranodal site

Data from A predictive model for aggressive non-Hodgkin's lymphoma. The International Non-Hodgkin's Lymphoma Prognostic Factors Project. N Engl J Med 1993;329(14):987–94.

</td></tr>
</table>

<table>
<tr><td>

Box 3
IPI survival rates

- Low risk (0–1 points): 5-year survival of 73%
- Low to intermediate risk (2 points): 5-year survival of 51%
- High to intermediate risk (3 points): 5-year survival of 43%
- High risk (4–5 points): 5-year survival of 26%

Data from A predictive model for aggressive non-Hodgkin's lymphoma. The International Non-Hodgkin's Lymphoma Prognostic Factors Project. N Engl J Med 1993;329(14):987–94.

</td></tr>
</table>

SUMMARY

Although the cause and molecular pathways of SS are still unknown, basic, clinical, and translational science have started to unravel what is occurring by identifying linkages to other known processes. With the advent of newer, more sensitive, and more accurate chemokine, cytokine, and genetic analysis, it is likely that the molecular progression of the disease will be understood. Even so, the modern technology of sialoendoscopy to treat obstructive sialoadenitis from mucous plugging, and the addition of rituximab to current chemotherapy, have allowed patients with SS to have a better quality of life and, if they develop lymphomatous changes, a significant increase in their disease remission and in their survival rate.

REFERENCES

1. Cobb BL, Lessard CJ, Harley JB, et al. Genes and Sjogren's syndrome. Rheum Dis Clin North Am 2008;34(4):847–68, vii.
2. Kassan SS, Moutsopoulos HM. Clinical manifestations and early diagnosis of Sjogren syndrome. Arch Intern Med 2004;164(12):1275–84.
3. Manthorpe R, Asmussen K, Oxholm P. Primary Sjogren's syndrome: diagnostic criteria, clinical features, and disease activity. J Rheumatol Suppl 1997;50:8–11.
4. Cruz-Tapias P, Rojas-Villarraga A, Maier-Moore S, et al. HLA and Sjogren's syndrome susceptibility. A meta-analysis of worldwide studies. Autoimmun Rev 2012;11(4):281–7.
5. Roitberg-Tambur A, Friedmann A, Safirman C, et al. Molecular analysis of HLA class II genes in primary Sjogren's syndrome. A study of Israeli Jewish and Greek non-Jewish patients. Hum Immunol 1993; 36(4):235–42.
6. Fridkis-Hareli M. Immunogenetic mechanisms for the coexistence of organ-specific and systemic autoimmune diseases. J Autoimmune Dis 2008;5:1.

7. Dawson L, Tobin A, Smith P, et al. Antimuscarinic antibodies in Sjogren's syndrome: where are we, and where are we going? Arthritis Rheum 2005;52(10): 2984–95.

8. Matsui M, Motomura D, Karasawa H, et al. Multiple functional defects in peripheral autonomic organs in mice lacking muscarinic acetylcholine receptor gene for the M3 subtype. Proc Natl Acad Sci U S A 2000;97(17):9579–84.

9. Nakamura T, Matsui M, Uchida K, et al. M(3) muscarinic acetylcholine receptor plays a critical role in parasympathetic control of salivation in mice. J Physiol 2004;558(Pt 2):561–75.

10. Kidd JF, Thorn P. Intracellular Ca2+ and Cl– channel activation in secretory cells. Annu Rev Physiol 2000; 62:493–513.

11. Wildenberg ME, van Helden-Meeuwsen CG, van de Merwe JP, et al. Systemic increase in type I interferon activity in Sjogren's syndrome: a putative role for plasmacytoid dendritic cells. Eur J Immunol 2008;38(7):2024–33.

12. Gottenberg JE, Cagnard N, Lucchesi C, et al. Activation of IFN pathways and plasmacytoid dendritic cell recruitment in target organs of primary Sjogren's syndrome. Proc Natl Acad Sci U S A 2006;103(8): 2770–5.

13. Gannot G, Lancaster HE, Fox PC. Clinical course of primary Sjogren's syndrome: salivary, oral, and serologic aspects. J Rheumatol Suppl 2000;27(8): 1905–9.

14. Dawson LJ, Smith PM, Moots RJ, et al. Sjogren's syndrome–time for a new approach. Rheumatology (Oxford) 2000;39(3):234–7.

15. Pederson T. Diffusional protein transport within the nucleus: a message in the medium. Nat Cell Biol 2000;2(5):E73–4.

16. Heft MW, Baum BJ. Unstimulated and stimulated parotid salivary flow rate in individuals of different ages. J Dent Res 1984;63(10):1182–5.

17. Ship JA, Nolan NE, Puckett SA. Longitudinal analysis of parotid and submandibular salivary flow rates in healthy, different-aged adults. J Gerontol A Biol Sci Med Sci 1995;50(5):M285–9.

18. Jonsson MV, Delaleu N, Brokstad KA, et al. Impaired salivary gland function in NOD mice: association with changes in cytokine profile but not with histopathologic changes in the salivary gland. Arthritis Rheum 2006;54(7):2300–5.

19. Dawson LJ, Stanbury J, Venn N, et al. Antimuscarinic antibodies in primary Sjogren's syndrome reversibly inhibit the mechanism of fluid secretion by human submandibular salivary acinar cells. Arthritis Rheum 2006;54(4):1165–73.

20. Waterman SA, Gordon TP, Rischmueller M. Inhibitory effects of muscarinic receptor autoantibodies on parasympathetic neurotransmission in Sjogren's syndrome. Arthritis Rheum 2000;43(7):1647–54.

21. Walker J, Gordon T, Lester S, et al. Increased severity of lower urinary tract symptoms and daytime somnolence in primary Sjogren's syndrome. J Rheumatol Suppl 2003;30(11):2406–12.

22. Bachmeyer C, Zuber M, Dupont S, et al. Adie syndrome as the initial sign of primary Sjogren syndrome. Am J Ophthalmol 1997;123(5):691–2.

23. Kovacs L, Torok T, Bari F, et al. Impaired microvascular response to cholinergic stimuli in primary Sjogren's syndrome. Ann Rheum Dis 2000;59(1):48–53.

24. Tumiati B, Perazzoli F, Negro A, et al. Heart rate variability in patients with Sjogren's syndrome. Clin Rheumatol 2000;19(6):477–80.

25. Bacman S, Sterin-Borda L, Camusso JJ, et al. Circulating antibodies against rat parotid gland M3 muscarinic receptors in primary Sjogren's syndrome. Clin Exp Immunol 1996;104(3):454–9.

26. Al-Hashimi I, Khuder S, Haghighat N, et al. Frequency and predictive value of the clinical manifestations in Sjogren's syndrome. J Oral Pathol Med 2001;30(1):1–6.

27. Vitali C, Bombardieri S, Jonsson R, et al. Classification criteria for Sjogren's syndrome: a revised version of the European criteria proposed by the American-European Consensus Group. Ann Rheum Dis 2002;61(6):554–8.

28. Shacham R, Puterman MB, Ohana N, et al. Endoscopic treatment of salivary glands affected by autoimmune diseases. J Oral Maxillofac Surg 2011;69(2):476–81.

29. Brook I. The bacteriology of salivary gland infections. Oral Maxillofacial Surg Clin N Am 2009; 21(3):269–74.

30. Bikker A. Increased expression of interleukin-7 in labial salivary glands of patients with primary Sjögren's syndrome correlates with increased inflammation. Arthritis Rheum 2010;62(4):969–77.

31. Brito-Zeron P, Ramos-Casals M, Nardi N, et al. Circulating monoclonal immunoglobulins in Sjogren syndrome: prevalence and clinical significance in 237 patients. Medicine 2005;84(2):90–7.

32. Voulgarelis M, Dafni UG, Isenberg DA, et al. Malignant lymphoma in primary Sjögren's syndrome: a multicenter, retrospective, clinical study by the European concerted action on Sjögren's syndrome. Arthritis Rheum 1999;42(8):1765–72.

33. Baimpa E, Dahabreh IJ, Voulgarelis M, et al. Hematologic manifestations and predictors of lymphoma development in primary Sjogren syndrome: clinical and pathophysiologic aspects. Medicine 2009; 88(5):284–93.

34. Voulgarelis M, Giannouli S, Ritis K, et al. Myelodysplasia-associated autoimmunity: clinical and pathophysiologic concepts. Eur J Clin Invest 2004; 34(10):690–700.

35. Voulgarelis M. B cell monoclonal proliferation in Sjogren's syndrome. Autoimmun Rev 2004;3(Suppl 1): S65–7.

36. Mariette X. Lymphomas complicating Sjogren's syndrome and hepatitis C virus infection may share a common pathogenesis: chronic stimulation of rheumatoid factor B cells. Ann Rheum Dis 2001;60(11):1007–10.

37. Rossi D, Gaidano G. Molecular heterogeneity of diffuse large B-cell lymphoma: implications for disease management and prognosis. Hematology 2002;7(4):239–52.

38. Neumeister P, Hoefler G, Beham-Schmid C, et al. Deletion analysis of the p16 tumor suppressor gene in gastrointestinal mucosa-associated lymphoid tissue lymphomas. Gastroenterology 1997;112(6):1871–5.

39. Routsias JG, Goules JD, Charalampakis G, et al. Malignant lymphoma in primary Sjogren's syndrome: an update on the pathogenesis and treatment. Semin Arthritis Rheum 2013;43(2):178–86.

40. A predictive model for aggressive non-Hodgkin's lymphoma. The International Non-Hodgkin's Lymphoma Prognostic Factors Project. N Engl J Med 1993;329(14):987–94.

41. Castrillo JM, Montalban C, Abraira V, et al. Evaluation of the international index in the prognosis of high grade gastric malt lymphoma. Leuk Lymphoma 1996;24(1–2):159–63.

42. Voulgarelis M, Ziakas PD, Papageorgiou A, et al. Prognosis and outcome of non-Hodgkin lymphoma in primary Sjogren syndrome. Medicine 2012; 91(1):1–9.

The Role of Parotidectomy in Sjögren's Syndrome

Rafael Madero-Visbal, MD, FACS[a], Zvonimir Milas, MD[b],*

KEYWORDS

- Xerophthalmia • Xerostomia • Non-Hodgkin lymphoma • Parotidectomy

KEY POINTS

- Sjögren's syndrome, a chronic and progressive autoimmune disorder mainly characterized by xerophthalmia, xerostomia, and parotid enlargement, is primarily managed medically, but some patients will require surgical management.
- Patients with Sjögren's syndrome have an increased risk of non-Hodgkin lymphoma. Superficial parotidectomy is indicated for diagnostic purposes and can be therapeutic in limited circumstances.
- Surgical indications for parotidectomy in Sjögren's syndrome include recurrent parotitis refractory to medical management; salivary gland malignancy; and severe, refractory pain.
- When indicated for recurrent bouts of parotitis, a total parotidectomy should be performed if possible.
- Surgical complications include transient or permanent facial nerve injury, post-operative pain, persistent inflammation of remnant parotid tissue, Frey syndrome, and facial scarring.

INTRODUCTION

In 1933, Dr. Henrik Sjögren originally described the triad of xerophthalmia (dry eyes), parotid enlargement, and arthritis. However, recognition of Sjögren's syndrome as an autoimmune process, both primary and secondary forms of presentation, did not occur until the 1960s.[1] Primary Sjögren's syndrome is mainly characterized by xerophthalmia and xerostomia (dry mouth), secondary to exocrine gland inflammation without any other connective tissue disorder.[2] Secondary Sjögren's syndrome is associated with other autoimmune diseases including scleroderma, rheumatoid arthritis, primary biliary cirrhosis, and systemic lupus erythematosus.[1–3]

Sjögren's syndrome is a chronic and progressive autoimmune disorder characterized by mononuclear cell infiltrate on exocrine glands, particularly of the periductal areas of the salivary and lacrimal glands. Most of the patients' symptomatology is directly related to salivary and lacrimal gland dysfunction secondary to B-Lymphocyte hyperreactivity, autoantibody production, and T-cell lymphocytic infiltration.[4] Consequently, the resultant clinical picture includes, most commonly, xerostomia, xerophthalmia, and parotid enlargement.[1–3,5] Upper airway and mucous-secreting gastrointestinal glands are less commonly involved exocrine organs and less likely symptomatic.[1,6]

In the United States, between $1/2$ million and 2 million patients are affected by Sjögren's syndrome, with an estimated prevalence of 1% to 3% in the general population.[1,7,8] Other studies have a wider range of population prevalence ranging from 0.1% to 4.8%. This discrepancy may be correlated to different genetic, environmental, geographic, and ethnic factors.[3,9,10] There is a 9:1 female-to-male ratio with disease peak of onset between the 4th and 6th decade of life. It is considered a slowly progressive and chronic

a MD Anderson Cancer Center, Orlando, 1400 S Orange Avenue, Orlando, FL 32806, USA; b Head and Neck Cancer Center, Levine Cancer Institute, UNC School of Medicine, Charlotte Campus, 1021 Morehead Medical Dr #3259, Charlotte, NC 28204, USA
* Corresponding author.
E-mail address: Zvonimir.Milas@carolinashealthcare.org

Oral Maxillofacial Surg Clin N Am 26 (2014) 83–90
http://dx.doi.org/10.1016/j.coms.2013.09.007
1042-3699/14/$ – see front matter © 2014 Elsevier Inc. All rights reserved.

disease; patients affected by Sjögren's syndrome have a much greater risk, up to 40-fold greater risk, of developing non-Hodgkin lymphoma than the general population.[1,3,4]

Sjögren's syndrome remains a disease treated primarily with medical management especially for the relief of symptoms. Surgical intervention is limited in its scope and indication. Although surgical procedures involving the parotid glands and the minor salivary glands are frequently performed for diagnostic purposes, superficial or total parotidectomies are uncommon for nonmalignant disease processes. However, there is a small group of Sjögren patients who derive a clinical benefit from parotidectomy for recurrent parotitis and other indications. In the following section, the authors discuss the indications, risks, and surgical technique for parotidectomy and other surgical interventions in patients with Sjögren's syndrome.

CLINICAL FINDINGS

Although Sjögren patients demonstrate a wide range of symptoms in the head and neck region, keratoconjunctivitis sicca or xerophthalmia is considered the hallmark clinical presentation. Together with xerostomia they describe the sicca complex.[3] Lacrimal gland and ocular surface immune inflammation leads to inadequate tear production, which results in corneal ulceration. These patients have symptoms such as ocular grittiness, blurring of vision, itchiness, and discomfort.[2,11,12] Salivary gland dysfunction, another classical symptom of Sjögren's syndrome, is most pertinent for expanded discussion as it results in clinical conditions that ultimately may lead to parotidectomy.

Xerostomia is the major consequence of gland dysfunction in the oral cavity, increasing the risk for dental cavities, premature tooth loss, dysphagia of solid foods, taste abnormalities, burning sensation, and changes in normal oral flora.[2,13–15] Early manifestations may include mild mucosal dryness, leading to smooth tongue with filiform papillae atrophy, angular cheilitis, and in some cases chronic erythematous candidiasis (thinning of mucosa with patchy mucosal erythema in palate or buccal mucosa).[3,5,16] Meanwhile, oral bruising or purpura has also been described in patients with Sjögren's syndrome–induced thrombocytopenia.[2,4]

Approximately, a third of patients with primary Sjögren's syndrome present with diffuse parotid gland enlargement induced by progressive lymphocyte infiltration.[6] Indeed, over the lifetime of patients with Sjögren's syndrome, as many as 80% of patients are thought to have parotid enlargement;[17] the majority are transitory or intermittent. Many patients also develop an infectious and inflammatory sialadenitis of the parotid gland, parotitis. The distortion of the parotid gland architecture from the autoimmune inflammatory infiltration predisposes Sjögren patients to parotitis. Medical therapy for parotitis includes antibiotics, sialogogues, nonsteroidal antiinflammatory drugs, and steroids. A culture swab of the purulent sialorrhea should be obtained from the buccal meatus of the duct to guide antibiotic choice. Gentle massage to express purulent sialorrhea and local heat are mechanical adjuncts to medical therapy. Chronic parotitis is characterized by recurrent episodes of painful parotid swelling with purulent sialorrhea. The treatment of chronic parotitis is the same as for acute parotitis, specifically medical management. However, when these episodes become too painful, too frequent, or poorly responsive to treatment, superficial or total parotidectomy should be considered.[17,18]

Another pertinent clinical presentation of Sjögren's syndrome that may lead to surgical intervention is the risk of developing non-Hodgkin lymphoma. Patients with primary or secondary Sjögren have a 44 times greater risk of developing lymphoma than the general population. Lymphoma tends to be a late occurrence in the natural history. The transformation initiates from polyclonal B lymphocytes activation to oligoclonal or monoclonal B-cell expansion that may result in a lymphoproliferative disorder.[3,6,19] Reported risk factors include type II mixed monoclonal cryoglobulinemia, palpable purpura, low C4 levels, splenomegaly, lymphadenopathy, and persistent parotid gland enlargement. Other extraglandular manifestations that may be associated with an increased risk of developing lymphoma include peripheral neuropathy, skin vasculitis, anemia, and lymphopenia. The majority of Sjögren-associated lymphomas are marginal zone B-cell lymphomas.[6] They are usually localized to the salivary glands, predominately in the parotid and submandibular glands, due to the chronic stimulation of autoreactive B cells leading to lymphomagenesis,[1] which frequently presents as a persistent parotid mass that increases in size. Given the significant rate of benign parotid enlargement, clinicians need to be vigilant in their evaluation and surveillance of parotid masses in Sjögren patients. The diagnosis of lymphoma usually begins with imaging for the identification of the parotid mass. The typical heterogeneity seen in grossly enlarged parotid glands, however, may hinder radiographic identification of small parotid masses. Following identification of the parotid mass on imaging, tissue diagnosis is required via fine-needle aspiration, core biopsy, or surgical biopsy and, if positive for lymphoma, a bone marrow biopsy for disease staging.[2]

DIAGNOSIS AND SURGERY

Sjögren's syndrome has a wide spectrum of clinical manifestation, requiring a high clinical suspicion for the detection and early management of the disease. The diagnosis is made by identifying previously established set of criteria based on signs and symptoms.[5,20] In 2002, the American-European Consensus Group designed an international set of diagnostic criteria for Sjögren's syndrome.[21–26] These set of criteria have a specificity of 97.2% and sensitivity of 48.6%.[3,21–23,27,28] They include oral and ocular symptoms, as well as laboratory findings. There are 6 overall criteria. Patients must present with at least 4 of the criteria with either positive labs or a positive salivary gland biopsy, a requisite for diagnosis (**Box 1**).[1,3,29] Exclusion criteria (**Box 2**) are identified as other conditions, and disease processes may mimic the symptoms of Sjögren's syndrome.

Oral manifestations of Sjögren's syndrome are evaluated by assessing salivary gland function and through salivary gland imaging. Salivary gland function is assessed by measuring secretion rate

---

Box 1
Inclusion criteria from the American-European Consensus Group

- Shirmer I test: positive (5 mm or less of wet strip in 5 min)[a]
- Salivary gland biopsy: focus score of 1 or higher (50 or more lymphocytes per 4 mm[2])[a]
- Ocular symptoms: subjective sense of dry eyes and/or use of tear substitute > 3x per day
- Oral symptoms: subjective sense of dry mouth, recurrent or persistent swollen salivary glands, and/or liquid substitute to assist food swallowing
- Ocular signs
- Rose Bengal or ocular dye score of 4 or more
- Positive salivary gland involvement determine by:
  - Salivary scintigraphy
  - Unstimulated salivary flow rate of 1.5 mL or less in 15 minutes
  - Parotid sialography with diffuse sialectasis
  - Anti-Ro Ag (SS-A) and/or Anti-La Ag (SS-B): positive

[a] First 2 criteria are requisite and mandatory for diagnosis.

Box 2
Exclusion conditions

- History of head and neck radiation treatment
- Hepatitis C infection
- Acquired immunodeficiency disease
- Preexisting lymphoma
- Sarcoidosis
- Graft-versus-host disease
- Current anticholinergic drug use

(sialometry) and analyzing salivary composition (sialochemistry).[11,12,30–32] Magnetic resonance imaging, computed tomography scanning, ultrasonography, scintigraphy, and sialography (exploration of gland ductal system) can all be used to image the parotid gland.[30] Each imaging modality has specific uses, strengths, and weaknesses, which is outside the scope of this discussion.

Salivary gland biopsies are performed to diagnose Sjögren's syndrome as seen earlier in the inclusion criteria. Parotid gland biopsies for diagnostic purposes are commonly performed through a 1- to 2-cm incision just below the ear-lobe around the posterior angle of the mandible. A small section of the superficial tail of the parotid is resected as this area has the least likelihood of injuring the facial nerve, cranial nerve (CN) VII. A reported complication, or rather risk, is permanent or transitory sensory loss around the preauricular incision area and inferior ear lobe.[33,34] The greater auricular nerve, the sensory nerve to this region, traverses the tail of the parotid and should be preserved if possible. Because of the risk of facial nerve injury, parotid biopsies have become infrequent. Another technique for diagnostic surgery is a labial minor salivary gland biopsy. The sensitivity varies from 63.5% to 93.7%, and the specificity is reported to be in excess of 89% in different studies.[29,33,35] Although a labial minor salivary gland is not without potential complications, these complications are usually less significant in magnitude in comparison to the complications of parotid gland biopsies. Reported complications from minor salivary gland biopsy include temporary or persistent paresthesias of the lower lip, pyogenic granulomas at the biopsy site, hematomas, cheloid formation, and local pain.[29,33,34,36,37] Surgical management is critical to establish diagnosis. The primary goal of these surgical biopsies is to obtain sufficient salivary gland tissue to identify focal lymphocytic infiltrates of the salivary glands, which are considered signs of target-organ specific damage in Sjögren's syndrome.[35,36]

MANAGEMENT OF SYMPTOMS AND SURGERY

The cornerstone in the treatment of patients with Sjögren's syndrome continues to be symptomatic relief; this is best achieved through a combination of local and systemic medical therapy, which ameliorates symptoms. Local control for xerophthalmia and xerostomia usually involves application of artificial tears and artificial salivary replacements, respectively, to relieve symptoms.[5,13,38] Systemic therapies can include pilocarpine (muscarinic M3 receptor agonist) or cevimeline (high-affinity M3 receptor agonist), which stimulate salivary flow.[38,39] Cyclosporine can also be used to increase salivary flow rate. Even electrical stimulation of the lingual nerve has been described to alleviate oral symptoms of pain and discomfort.[1,3] Still other patients respond to more systemic agents like corticosteroids, plaquenil, azathioprine, methotrexate, intravenous immunoglobulins, rituximab, and mycophenolate mophetil.[3,4,40,41] Certain patients with early or nonrecurrent sialadenitis of the parotid may benefit from more invasive techniques such as parotid sialendoscopy with ductal rinsing and even Stenson duct dilation. Parotidectomy, for benign disease, is most often performed once all other local and systemic options have been attempted.

Indications for Parotidectomy

Parotid gland involvement in patients with Sjögren's syndrome can lead to chronic gland swelling, infection, and malignant transformation as described above. The most common indication for parotidectomy is to identify salivary gland–based malignancy. In some patients with Sjögren's syndrome, parotid gland enlargement is transitory, infectious in others, and chronic in still others. However, the dramatically increased risk of lymphoma dictates close clinical and radiographic surveillance in patients with parotid enlargement for prompt and accurate diagnosis.[38,39] Patients with Sjögren's syndrome are 44 times more likely to develop non-Hodgkin lymphoma as well as a significantly increased risk to develop Waldenström macroglobulinemia than the general population.[17,42,43] Fine-needle aspiration of parotid masses is used to make a diagnosis. The diagnostic accuracy of fine-needle aspiration or core biopsy of the parotid gland is at best 80% for all parotid lesions.[44] However, there is a significant diagnostic challenge on fine-needle aspiration to differentiate between a lymphoma and a benign Sjögren's syndrome lymphocytic inflammatory infiltration of the parotid gland. Deep incisional biopsies of the parotid gland are not recommended because of the risk facial nerve injury. Thus, suspicious parotid masses identified clinically and on surveillance imaging are clear indications for a superficial parotidectomy for diagnosis.

Parotidectomy can also be considered therapeutic for early-stage lymphoma, which is limited to the parotid only and has a low-grade histology, specifically mucosa-associated lymphoid tissue (MALT)/marginal zone (MZ) non-Hodgkin lymphoma. Patients with MALT/MZ histology often have several options between therapeutic modalities, specifically systemic chemotherapy, radiation therapy, and surgery for early-stage disease of the parotid.[45] Although radiation therapy is often effective for lymphoma, the side effects of radiation therapy in patients with Sjögren's syndrome can severely exacerbate the xerostomia from which patients already suffer. Furthermore, the radiation therapy's negative effects on oral health and dentition can also be potentiated in this patient population. Early-stage MALT/MZ non-Hodgkin lymphoma can be managed with surgery when the disease is limited to the parotid and is surgically resectable without significant complication. Surgical intent must be tempered based on the extent of tumoral involvement. Aggressive surgery with facial nerve sacrifice is contraindicated given the systemic nature of lymphoma and the role of chemotherapy and radiation in its treatment.[46] Also, there is no role for parotidectomy if the patient has systemic disease and a diagnosis of lymphoma has already been established by other means.

Recurrent parotitis refractory to medical management or with intractable pain meets criteria for surgical intervention. Recurrent parotitis can also lead to parotid abscesses, which may need to be incised and drained carefully. Ideally, the patient should be managed through the acute infectious phase of the disease and be given an opportunity to clinically resolve before a parotidectomy is performed.[17] There is a paucity of literature, which describes the extent of surgical resection required for chronic parotitis. The best literature was published several decades ago. The lack of more contemporary literature may reflect not only the infrequency of this procedure but also the effectiveness of medical management and medical advances in the management of the immune component of Sjögren's syndrome. Total parotidectomy with sparring of the facial nerve is generally recommended by the investigators as it minimizes the risk of remnant deep lobe parotid tissue to continue the cycle of swelling and infection.[17,18,42] Their recommendations are based on the observation that any remnant parotid gland tissue may be a target for recurrent autoimmune or infectious pathology.[17,18] Indeed, patients with Sjögren's syndrome are more likely to present with surgical wound complications, especially with a remnant deep parotid lobe, including recurrent infections and salivary fistulas.[42] The chronic inflammation from recurrent parotitis also increases the difficulty of facial nerve dissection and the risk of facial nerve paralysis.[18] Thus, recurrent, chronic parotitis is an indication for parotidectomy, but it is associated with increased complications and should be considered only when medical options fail.

Parotidectomy is also considered to address the chronic parotid enlargement that affects these patients' quality of life, aesthetic presentation, and facial pain/discomfort. The majority of patients have parotid enlargement at some point in the natural history of their disease. Medical therapy should be the primary modality of treatment to which most patients respond. But when patients with Sjögren's syndrome have refractory glandular enlargement and chronic pain, which interferes with daily social function, surgical resection of the parotid can help. Post-operative exacerbation of xerostomia is a concern. However, the disease process at this point usually has damaged the gland and patients already present with significant degrees of xerostomia. In this setting, the xerostomia side effects from the surgical intervention become negligible.[17,18,42] The surgeon and the patient should have a thorough discussion to discuss the risk/benefit ratio of parotidectomy.

Anatomic and Technical Considerations

The parotid gland is the largest salivary gland and is divided into a deep and superficial lobe connected by an isthmus in the middle. CN VII, the facial nerve, lies anterior to the isthmus and provides the anatomic division between these lobes. The facial nerve provides innervation to the muscles of mimetic function. The parotid gland is enveloped by the parotidomasseteric fascia, a deep cervical fascia derivative. Although the base of the parotid gland lies on the zygomatic arch, its apex is posterior to the mandible's angle. Stensen's duct (the parotid duct) extends from the base of the earlobe to the vermilion border of the upper lip. The duct is anteromedial to the masseter muscle anterior border, and it transverses the buccinator muscle before entering the oral cavity opposite to the second maxillary molar. Embedded within the gland, and superficial to the deep plane, are the parotid plexus, the facial nerve and branches, the retromandibular vein, and the external carotid artery.[47–51]

Identification of the facial nerve is a critical component of any surgery involving the parotid gland. The motor component of the facial nerve innervates muscle of face expression, scalp, buccinators, platysma, stylohyoid, posterior belly of digastric, external ear, and stapedius. Meanwhile, the sensory components of the facial nerve innervates the anterior two-thirds of the tongue and supplies sensation to the external acoustic meatus, soft palate, and pharynx. Thus, injury to the facial nerve at the extracranial/intraparotid level can have significant functional outcome. The facial nerve leaves the stylomastoid foramen entering the parotid gland. The pes anserinus is the branch point for the facial nerve where it divides into 2 primary branches, the cervicofacial and temporozygomatic branches, within the parotid gland at the posterior border of the mandible ramus (**Fig. 1**). The temporozygomatic branch of the facial nerve lies between the superficial and deep lobe, just above the gland's isthmus.[47,50–52]

Among the surgical techniques described, the modified Blair incision (**Fig. 2**) is the most commonly used technique to access the parotid gland, because the less visible scar is cosmetically advantageous for the patient.[53–56] There are several mechanisms to identify the facial nerve during surgical procedures to preserve its integrity. The surgical landmarks most widely described include the tympanomastoid suture, the styloid process, the tragal pointer, the posterior belly of the digastric muscle, and the transverse process of the axis. The tympanomastoid suture is the most reliable anatomic structure. Typically, the facial nerve is localized 2 to 4 mm deep to the medial end of the structure, which leads directly to the stylomastoid foramen. The posterior belly of the digastric muscle is also very useful for the identification of the nerve. As the posterior belly of the digastric muscle approaches its insertion, the nerve is identified just superior to the belly.[47,49–52]

Complications

The most feared complication of superficial or total parotid surgery is facial nerve damage because it is both a functional and a cosmetically visible injury. Although transient deficit has been reported in 20% to 40% of cases, permanent dysfunction has been found in 0% to 4% of cases.[18,52,55,57] As described earlier, patients with recurrent parotitis and chronic inflammation of the gland have a slightly increased risk for facial nerve injury. To avoid this complication, passive electrophysiologic nerve monitoring is used to record electromyographic signals from the facial muscles through needle electrodes on the skin. Monitoring

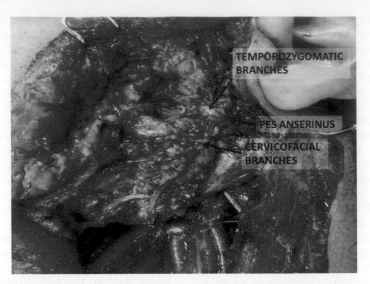

Fig. 1. Facial nerve.

the nerves allows the surgeon to help identify and preserve the facial nerve, especially in inflamed and scarred parotid tissue. The areas innervated by the facial nerve that are mainly monitored are the frontal, zygomatic, buccal, and marginal mandibular areas.[47–50,54–58]

Although short- and/or long-term facial nerve paralysis is the most concerning complication of parotidectomy, other negative outcomes have been widely described including pain, loss of sensation, gustatory sweating (auriculotemporal or Frey syndrome), and facial scarring with possible keloid formation. Furthermore, cases of

salivary fistula formation, auricular nerve anesthesia, wound infections; hematoma, and seroma have also been reported.[55–57,59] Meticulous surgical techniques play a major role in avoiding these complications, for example, a modified face-lift incision, suggested by Terris and colleagues, instead of a modified Blair incision will minimize face scarring.[57,59]

SUMMARY

Sjögren's syndrome is a chronic and progressive autoimmune disorder mainly characterized by xerophthalmia, xerostomia, and parotid enlargement. Although the cornerstone for treatment consists of medical management, a small percentage of patients require surgical intervention. More limited surgical procedures are important for the diagnosis and occasionally the symptomatic management of Sjögren's syndrome. Indications for parotidectomy in patients with Sjögren's syndrome are relatively narrow. Because patients have an increased risk of developing non-Hodgkin lymphoma, parotidectomy is often necessary for diagnosis of parotid lesions. Other indications for parotidectomy include recurrent parotitis that is refractory to medical management and in patients with intractable pain of the parotid. Total parotidectomy is recommended for the complete removal of salivary tissue in patients with recurrent parotitis. There is an increased risk of injury to the nerve, reflecting the difficulty in identification and dissection in a chronically inflamed organ. Although medical management is the mainstay of treatment, a cohort of patients benefit greatly from parotidectomy for appropriate indications.

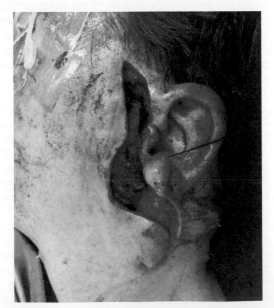

Fig. 2. Modified Blair incision.

REFERENCES

1. Mahoney EJ, Spiegel JH. Sjogren's disease. Otolaryngol Clin North Am 2003;36(4):733–45.
2. Carr AJ, Ng WF, Figueiredo F, et al. Sjogren's syndrome - an update for dental practitioners. Br Dent J 2012;213(7):353–7.
3. Peri Y, Agmon-Levin N, Theodor E, et al. Sjogren's syndrome, the old and the new. Best Pract Res Clin Rheumatol 2012;26(1):105–17.
4. Al-Hashimi I. Sjogren's syndrome: diagnosis and management. Womens Health (Lond Engl) 2007; 3(1):107–22.
5. Mays JW, Sarmadi M, Moutsopoulos NM. Oral manifestations of systemic autoimmune and inflammatory diseases: diagnosis and clinical management. J Evid Based Dent Pract 2012;12(3 Suppl):265–82.
6. Tucci M, Quatraro C, Silvestris F. Sjogren's syndrome: an autoimmune disorder with otolaryngological involvement. Acta Otorhinolaryngol Ital 2005;25(3):139–44.
7. Liew MS, Zhang M, Kim E, et al. Provalence and predictors of Sjogren's syndrome in a prospective cohort of patients with aqueous-deficient dry eye. Br J Ophthalmol 2012;96(12):1498–503.
8. Sanchez-Guerrero J, Perez-Dosal MR, Cardenas-Velazquez F, et al. Prevalence of Sjogren's syndrome in ambulatory patients according to the American-European Consensus Group criteria. Rheumatology (Oxford) 2005;44(2):235–40.
9. Kessel A, Toubi E, Rozenbaum M, et al. Sjogren's syndrome in the community: can serology replace salivary gland biopsy? Rheumatol Int 2006;26(4): 337–9.
10. Segal B, Bowman SJ, Fox PC, et al. Primary Sjogren's Syndrome: health experiences and predictors of health quality among patients in the United States. Health Qual Life Outcomes 2009;7:46.
11. Vissink A, Bootsma H, Spijkervet FK, et al. Current and future challenges in primary Sjogren's syndrome. Curr Pharm Biotechnol 2012;13(10): 2026–45.
12. Vissink A, Kalk WW, Mansour K, et al. Comparison of lacrimal and salivary gland involvement in Sjogren's syndrome. Arch Otolaryngol Head Neck Surg 2003;129(9):966–71.
13. Stewart CM, Berg KM, Cha S, et al. Salivary dysfunction and quality of life in Sjogren syndrome: a critical oral-systemic connection. J Am Dent Assoc 2008;139(3):291–9.
14. Enger TB, Palm O, Garen T, et al. Oral distress in primary Sjogren's syndrome: implications for health-related quality of life. Eur J Oral Sci 2011; 119(6):474–80.
15. Castro I, Sepulveda D, Cortes J, et al. Oral dryness in Sjogren's syndrome patients. Not just a question of water. Autoimmun Rev 2013;12(5):567–74.
16. Fox PC, Bowman SJ, Segal B, et al. Oral involvement in primary Sjogren syndrome. J Am Dent Assoc 2008;139(12):1592–601.
17. Bone RC, Fox RI, Howell FV, et al. Sjogren's syndrome: a persistent clinical problem. Laryngoscope 1985;95(3):295–9.
18. Arriaga MA, Myers EN. The surgical management of chronic parotitis. Laryngoscope 1990;100(12): 1270–5.
19. Zenone T. Parotid gland non-Hodgkin lymphoma in primary Sjogren syndrome. Rheumatol Int 2012; 32(5):1387–90.
20. Galvez J, Saiz E, Lopez P, et al. Diagnostic evaluation and classification criteria in Sjogren's Syndrome. Joint Bone Spine 2009;76(1):44–9.
21. Vitali C, Bootsma H, Bowman SJ, et al. Classification criteria for Sjogren's syndrome: we actually need to definitively resolve the long debate on the issue. Ann Rheum Dis 2013;72(4):476–8.
22. Seror R, Ravaud P, Mariette X, et al. EULAR Sjogren's Syndrome Patient Reported Index (ESSPRI): development of a consensus patient index for primary Sjogren's syndrome. Ann Rheum Dis 2011; 70(6):968–72.
23. Seror R, Ravaud P, Bowman SJ, et al. EULAR Sjogren's syndrome disease activity index: development of a consensus systemic disease activity index for primary Sjogren's syndrome. Ann Rheum Dis 2010;69(6):1103–9.
24. Bowman SJ, Booth DA, Platts RG, et al. Validation of the Sicca Symptoms Inventory for clinical studies of Sjogren's syndrome. J Rheumatol 2003; 30(6):1259–66.
25. Bowman SJ. Collaborative research into outcome measures in Sjogren's syndrome. Update on disease assessment. Scand J Rheumatol Suppl 2002;116:23–7.
26. Bowman SJ, Pillemer S, Jonsson R, et al. Revisiting Sjogren's syndrome in the new millennium: perspectives on assessment and outcome measures. Report of a workshop held on 23 March 2000 at Oxford, UK. Rheumatology (Oxford) 2001;40(10):1180–8.
27. Seror R, Gottenberg JE, Devauchelle-Pensec V, et al. ESSDAI and ESSPRI: EULAR indexes for a complete picture of primary Sjogren's syndrome patients. Arthritis Care Res (Hoboken) 2013;65:1358–64.
28. Seror R, Bootsma H, Bowman SJ, et al. Outcome measures for primary Sjogren's syndrome. J Autoimmun 2012;39(1–2):97–102.
29. Guellec D, Cornec D, Jousse-Joulin S, et al. Diagnostic value of labial minor salivary gland biopsy for Sjogren's syndrome: a systematic review. Autoimmun Rev 2013;12(3):416–20.
30. Kalk WW, Vissink A, Spijkervet FK, et al. Parotid sialography for diagnosing Sjogren syndrome. Oral Surg Oral Med Oral Pathol Oral Radiol Endod 2002;94(1):131–7.

31. Gotoh S, Watanabe Y, Fujibayashi T. Validity of stimulated whole saliva collection as a sialometric evaluation for diagnosing Sjogren's syndrome. Oral Surg Oral Med Oral Pathol Oral Radiol Endod 2005;99(3):299–302.

32. Fabijanic I, Markeljevic J, Markov-Glavas D. Fine-needle aspiration cytology, salivary gland ultrasonography, and sialography in the evaluation of primary Sjogren's syndrome. Scand J Rheumatol 2006;35(1):77–8.

33. Colella G, Cannavale R, Vicidomini A, et al. Salivary gland biopsy: a comprehensive review of techniques and related complications. Rheumatology (Oxford) 2010;49(11):2117–21.

34. Pijpe J, Kalk WW, van der Wal JE, et al. Parotid gland biopsy compared with labial biopsy in the diagnosis of patients with primary Sjogren's syndrome. Rheumatology (Oxford) 2007;46(2):335–41.

35. Bamba R, Sweiss NJ, Langerman AJ, et al. The minor salivary gland biopsy as a diagnostic tool for Sjogren syndrome. Laryngoscope 2009;119(10):1922–6.

36. Salomonsson S, Rozell BL, Heimburger M, et al. Minor salivary gland immunohistology in the diagnosis of primary Sjogren's syndrome. J Oral Pathol Med 2009;38(3):282–8.

37. Obinata K, Sato T, Ohmori K, et al. A comparison of diagnostic tools for Sjogren syndrome, with emphasis on sialography, histopathology, and ultrasonography. Oral Surg Oral Med Oral Pathol Oral Radiol Endod 2010;109(1):129–34.

38. Mavragani CP, Moutsopoulos NM, Moutsopoulos HM. The management of Sjogren's syndrome. Nat Clin Pract Rheumatol 2006;2(5):252–61.

39. Mavragani CP, Moutsopoulos HM. Conventional therapy of Sjogren's syndrome. Clin Rev Allergy Immunol 2007;32(3):284–91.

40. Pijpe J, Meijer JM, Bootsma H, et al. Clinical and histologic evidence of salivary gland restoration supports the efficacy of rituximab treatment in Sjogren's syndrome. Arthritis Rheum 2009;60(11):3251–6.

41. Pijpe J, van Imhoff GW, Vissink A, et al. Changes in salivary gland immunohistology and function after rituximab monotherapy in a patient with Sjogren's syndrome and associated MALT lymphoma. Ann Rheum Dis 2005;64(6):958–60.

42. Rosen IB, McHenry CR, Bedard YC. Surgical treatment in non-neoplastic parotid disease: indications and results. Can J Surg 1992;35(5):560–4.

43. Kristinsson SY, Koshiol J, Bjorkholm M, et al. Immune-related and inflammatory conditions and risk of lymphoplasmacytic lymphom or Waldenstrom macroglobulinemia. J Natl Cancer Inst 2010;102(8):557–67.

44. Burke C, Thomas R, Inglis C, et al. Ultrasound-guided core biopsy in the diagnosis of lymphoma of the head and neck. A 9 year experience. Br J Radiol 2011;84(1004):727–32.

45. Hitchcock S, Ng AK, Fisher DC, et al. Treatment outcome of mucosa-associated lymphoid tissue/marginal zone non-Hodgkin's lymphoma. Int J Radiat Oncol Biol Phys 2002;52(4):1058–66.

46. Feinstein AJ, Ciarleglio MM, Cong X, et al. Parotid gland lymphoma: prognostic analysis of 2140 patients. Laryngoscope 2013;123(5):1199–203.

47. Wang SJ, Eisele DW. Parotidectomy–Anatomical considerations. Clin Anat 2012;25(1):12–8.

48. Bova R, Saylor A, Coman WB. Parotidectomy: review of treatment and outcomes. ANZ J Surg 2004;74(7):563–8.

49. Pericot J, Monner A, Piulachs P, et al. Parotidectomy technique in the treatment of parotid tumours (an analysis of 70 cases). J Maxillofac Surg 1982;10(1):35–41.

50. Bailey H. Parotidectomy: indications and results. Br Med J 1947;1(4499):404–7.

51. Singh RP, Abdel-Galil K, Harbottle M, et al. Parotid gland disease in childhood: diagnosis and indications for surgical intervention. Br J Oral Maxillofac Surg 2012;50(4):338–43.

52. Plopper C, Cernea CR, Ferraz AR, et al. Parotidectomy for primary nonparotid diseases. Otolaryngol Head Neck Surg 2004;131(4):407–12.

53. Schultz PW, Woods JE. Subtotal parotidectomy in the treatment of chronic sialadenitis. Ann Plast Surg 1983;11(6):459–61.

54. Powell ME, Clairmont AA. Complications of parotidectomy. South Med J 1983;76(9):1109–12.

55. Moeller K, Esser D, Boeger D, et al. Parotidectomy and submandibulectomy for benign diseases in Thuringia, Germany: a population-based study on epidemiology and outcome. Eur Arch Otorhinolaryngol 2013;270(3):1149–55.

56. Guntinas-Lichius O, Klussmann JP, Wittekindt C, et al. Parotidectomy for benign parotid disease at a university teaching hospital: outcome of 963 operations. Laryngoscope 2006;116(4):534–40.

57. Nitzan D, Kronenberg J, Horowitz Z, et al. Quality of life following parotidectomy for malignant and benign disease. Plast Reconstr Surg 2004;114(5):1060–7.

58. Maddox PT, Paydarfar JA, Davies L. Parotidectomy: a 17-year institutional experience at a rural academic medical center. Ann Otol Rhinol Laryngol 2012;121(2):100–3.

59. Grover N, D'Souza A. Facelift approach for parotidectomy: an evolving aesthetic technique. Otolaryngol Head Neck Surg 2013;148(4):548–56.

Extraglandular Manifestations of Primary Sjögren's Syndrome

Sabatino Ienopoli, DO[a,b], Steven E. Carsons, MD[a,b],*

KEYWORDS

- Sjögren's syndrome • Extraglandular • Vasculitis • Arthropathy

KEY POINTS

- As many as 50% of patients with primary Sjögren's syndrome may experience extraglandular symptoms.
- Musculoskeletal symptoms include arthralgia and mild inflammatory arthritis, and myalgia.
- Neurologic involvement may occur in up to 20%. Peripheral neuropathy is fairly common; central nervous system involvement is rare.
- Respiratory symptoms reflect involvement of the upper airway with sicca manifestations, such as dry nose and dry cough; lower respiratory tract involvement usually involves interstitial lung disease.
- Vasculitis most often presents with palpable purpura and may be associated with risk for non-Hodgkin lymphoma.

Sjögren's syndrome is a chronic autoimmune disease that typically affects the salivary and lacrimal glands. It is also described as a lymphoinfiltrative disorder that affects exocrine glands producing dry eyes and dry mouth. Aside from the common glandular signs and symptoms, Sjögren's syndrome may also cause mononuclear infiltration and immune complex deposition involving extraglandular sites producing several extraglandular manifestations (EGMs) (**Box 1**). The prevalence of EGMs varies greatly depending on the particular manifestation. In some studies, EGMs are quite prevalent. For instance, in a report by Hernandez-Molina and colleagues[1] examining 109 patients with primary Sjögren's syndrome (pSS), 86% had at least one EGM. In this article we look at the ways that EGM may present in patients with pSS (see **Box 1**). The focus is specifically on the more prevalent and significant EGMs including involvement the nervous system, pulmonary manifestations, vasculitis associated with pSS, and arthropathy.

NERVOUS SYSTEM
Peripheral Nervous System

The prevalence of peripheral neuropathy in pSS has been reported to be anywhere from 2% to 60% in the literature (**Box 2**). The wide range reported is likely caused by the classification criteria used by the various studies and the criteria used to define neuropathy. Some reports used clinical symptoms with less objective inclusion criteria, whereas others relied on definitive criteria, such as nerve conduction studies.

The cause of peripheral neuropathy secondary to pSS is yet to be fully understood. Some have thought it because of vasculitis of the peripheral

a Division of Rheumatology, Allergy and Immunology, Department of Medicine, Winthrop University Hospital, Stony Brook School of Medicine, 120 Mineola Boulevard, Suite 410, Mineola NY 11501, USA; b State University of New York at Stony Brook School of Medicine, Stony Brook, NY 11794, USA
* Corresponding author. Division of Rheumatology, Allergy and Immunology, Department of Medicine, Winthrop University Hospital, Stony Brook School of Medicine, 120 Mineola Boulevard, Suite 410, Mineola NY 11501, USA.
E-mail address: scarsons@winthrop.org

Oral Maxillofacial Surg Clin N Am 26 (2014) 91–99
http://dx.doi.org/10.1016/j.coms.2013.09.008
1042-3699/14/$ – see front matter © 2014 Elsevier Inc. All rights reserved.

Box 1
Reported EGMs of primary Sjögren's syndrome

Peripheral neuropathy[a]

Central nervous system involvement[a]

Trigeminal neuralgia[a]

Autonomic neuropathy[a]

Dementia/confusion[a]

Pancreatitis

Gastroparesis

Autoimmune hepatitis

Primary biliary cirrhosis

Tubulointerstitial nephritis

Cough[a]

Dyspnea[a]

Sinusitis[a]

Septal perforation[a]

Interstitial lung disease[a]

Vasculitis[a]

Arthralgias[a]

Arthritis[a]

Lymphoma

Amyloidosis

Fibromyalgia[a]

Raynaud phenomenon

   [a] Discussed in further in detail.

nerves.[2] Dorsal root ganglionitis with degeneration of dorsal root ganglion neurons and mononuclear cell infiltration without true vasculitis has been associated with the sensory ataxic form of

Box 2
Neurologic involvement

- Patients experiencing peripheral neuropathy associated with Sjögren's syndrome can present in multiple ways including abnormal vibratory sensation, impaired position sense, parethesias, and weakness.

- Central nervous system involvement in pSS can closely mimic multiple sclerosis. Clinical history, lumbar puncture, and magnetic resonance imaging findings may help differentiate the two.

- Patients with pSS have reported low mood, decreased quality of life, and impaired concentration, which can be significantly improved if addressed by supportive measures.

Sjögren's syndrome–associated neuropathy.[3,4] Peripheral neuropathy is a term that seems to encompass a diverse subset of specific neuropathies associated with pSS as described next.

Sensory Ataxic Neuropathy

This form of neuropathy is caused by a lesion in the dorsal root ganglia and can involve all sensory modalities. Although this type of neuropathy can be seen with Sjögren's syndrome it is most commonly associated with paraneoplastic syndrome.[5] Other etiologies to consider when encountering this type of neuropathy are pyridoxine toxicity, human T-lymphotropic virus-1 infection, and HIV infection.[5] It is reported that patients with Sjögren's syndrome with this type of neuropathy do not have other prominent EGMs. The timing of the onset of the first symptom to its full-blown picture is typically months to years. It has been reported as mostly asymmetric in presentation.[2] On examination there are abnormal findings in vibratory sensation and impaired position sense, a positive Romberg sign, and absent deep tendon reflexes.[2,4,6] In one study examining 36 patients with this form of neuropathy, all were found to display pseudoathetosis.[2] Muscle strength is spared until late stages of the process when it begins to noticeably lessen.

Axonal Sensorimotor Polyneuropathy

This type of neuropathy usually presents with distal paresthesias and sensory deficits that are similar to other types of sensory neuropathy. The muscle weakness that accompanies the sensory deficits is also usually distal and also symmetric in distribution.[7] On physical examination, deep tendon reflexes are usually diminished or absent.[8]

Trigeminal Neuralgia

Patients with Sjögren's syndrome with trigeminal neuralgia may present either unilaterally or bilaterally and typically report numbness or paraesthesia.[2] Motor symptoms have not been reported in trigeminal neuralgia associated with Sjögren's syndrome. Fifteen patients studied were found to have a pure sensory neuropathy.[2]

Autonomic Neuropathy

Autonomic neuropathy is thought to be rare in Sjögren's syndrome but may be underreported. In a study examining 92 patients with pSS-associated neuropathy only three were found to have autonomic neuropathy. These patients were found to have Adie pupil (a dilated pupil that does not constrict to light); orthostatic hypotension with syncope; abdominal pain; constipation; and diarrhea. Hypohidrosis or anhidrosis involving the trunk and all four limbs may occur.[2] Urinary symptoms may also be present.

Central Nervous System Involvement

pSS with central nervous system (CNS) involvement can manifest in a variety of ways including transverse myelitis, optic neuropathy, hemiparesis, transient ischemic attacks, and movement or cognitive dysfunction. The prevalence of pSS with CNS involvement has been reported to be as high as 20%, but most estimates are lower and in the range of 2% to 10%.[9–11] Alexander and colleagues[11] studied 20 patients with pSS and CNS involvement. The average age of onset of CNS disease was 38 years of age, whereas the mean time for the diagnosis of pSS was 42 years of age. This may be because the subgroup with CNS disease could represent an overlap syndrome. One CNS disease that has been reported to occur in association with Sjögren's syndrome is multiple sclerosis (MS). Patients with pSS can suffer from a multifocal CNS disease with either a relapsing or progressive course similar to the presentation seen with MS.[12] MS and pSS are autoimmune disorders with a tendency to predominate in women. In a study by de Seze and colleagues,[13] who studied 60 patients with primary progressive MS, 10 patients (16.7%) met criteria for Sjögren's syndrome using the European community study group on diagnostic criteria for Sjögren's syndrome.[14] Considering that the prevalence of Sjögren's syndrome may be between 1% and 5% it is important to consider the differential diagnosis of Sjögren's syndrome when considering a diagnosis of MS. Although CNS symptoms may be similar in the two disease states, Sjögren's syndrome can be differentiated by symptoms and objective evidence of the sicca complex, the presence of vasculitis involving the skin and muscle, peripheral neuropathy, cognitive changes occurring at the early stages, and serologic abnormalities specific for Sjögren's syndrome (SS-A, SS-B).[12]

A lumbar puncture is commonly performed as a diagnostic test for MS and should be performed should CNS Sjögren's be suspected. In a study of 20 patients with pSS and CNS disease, cerebrospinal fluid analysis showed elevated total protein, IgG index, a mononuclear pleocytosis of mainly lymphoid cells, and oligoclonal bands.[11] These results are similar to those found in patients with MS; however, although oligoclonal bands can be seen in patients with both etiologies there is a difference in the quantity seen. Patients with MS were found to have multiple bands, whereas patients with pSS typically had one to two bands present.[11]

It has been frequently reported that patients with pSS have an increase in CNS lesions.[15–18] Patients with pSS may have an increase in white matter hyperintensities in the subcortical and periventricular white matter on T2-weighted and FLAIR images.[16]

The immunopathology of CNS involvement in pSS has yet to be fully understood. Histopathologic examination of brain tissue from some patients with pSS and CNS involvement has shown small-vessel mononuclear inflammatory and ischemic-hemorrhagic vasculopathy.[19]

Psychiatric Involvement

Psychiatric involvement has also been associated with pSS. In a series of articles by Valtysdottir and colleagues[20] it was reported that patients with pSS have been found to exhibit more anxiety and depression compared with patients who have rheumatoid arthritis (RA). They were also observed to complain more frequently of low mood, impaired concentration, and gastrointestinal disturbances. Using the Psychological General Well Being Index, patients with pSS were found to have a lower sense of well-being and decreased quality of life compared with patients with RA.[20] These articles shed light on an area that may be overlooked when treating patients with pSS. Although the sicca complex tends to be the area of focus for Sjögren's syndrome, a physician must consider the whole patient and in doing so screen for depression. Quality of life in patients with pSS may be significantly improved if such topics as anxiety, depression, and overall mood are addressed.

Cognitive impairment and dementia have also been reported in pSS. Although prospective studies have not been reported, there have been numerous case studies attributing a form of dementia to SS. Although rare, physicians may need to consider pSS as a possible cause for such symptoms.

pSS is a common autoimmune disease in patients older than age 50. Although mainly viewed as a glandular disease producing the hallmark features of dry eyes and dry mouth, it should be recognized that pSS frequently includes EGMs including the nervous system. The prevalence of peripheral neuropathy seen in pSS and the variety of subtypes by which it may present should remind the physician to conduct a thorough and complete neurologic examination when examining a patient with pSS. Although not yet as well documented as peripheral nervous system disease, CNS involvement related to pSS may affect the physical and psychological aspect of a patient's life. Quality of life and dementia are areas of pSS that require further study.

Pulmonary Involvement

Pulmonary involvement has been reported to involve anywhere from 9% to 75% of patients with pSS (**Box 3**).[21,22] This wide range is likely caused by differences in the criteria used to classify cases of pSS and in the case definitions of pulmonary involvement. A study done by Yazisiz and colleagues[23] reported an 11.4% prevalence of pulmonary involvement based on radiologic findings, whereas a study by Constantopoulos and colleagues[22] reported a prevalence of 75% when using clinical symptoms or histologic data.

The clinical manifestations of pulmonary Sjögren's syndrome may be subtle at the time of presentation. Although cough seems to be the most common pulmonary manifestation, dyspnea on exertion, chest pain, and wheeze also have been frequently reported. A nonspecific symptom, such as cough, may be difficult to recognize as the presenting sign of pulmonary involvement in Sjögren's syndrome. Cough presents a wide differential diagnostic spectrum, and this may significantly delay medical attention and ultimately an underestimation of its prevalence. Papiris and colleagues[24] studied 61 patients with pSS and found that 41% were found to have dry cough as the main pulmonary symptom. This nonproductive cough seen in many patients with pSS has often been described as "bronchitis sicca" and thought to be caused by desiccation of the mucosa of the tracheobronchial tree.[24]

Box 3
Pulmonary involvement

- The most common symptoms are cough and dyspnea on exertion.
- Nonspecific symptoms, such as cough and dyspnea, may delay recognition as an EGM of pSS allowing further damage to occur before being properly treated.
- Lymphocytic interstitial pneumonitis, nonspecific interstitial pneumonia, and usual interstitial pneumonia may occur in patients with pSS and without appropriate treatment can lead to permanent lung pathology.
- Pulmonary involvement and pSS has been associated with a fourfold increase in mortality in 10 years compared with patients with pSS without pulmonary involvement.

Because of decreased glandular function accompanying Sjögren's syndrome, dryness of the upper airway commonly occurs. This can lead to such symptoms as bleeding, sinusitis, septal perforation, or taste and smell disturbances.[25] Xerotrachea (dryness of the mucosa of the trachea) is reported to affect 17% of patients with pSS and also may present as a nonproductive cough.[22] In a study by Papiris and colleagues[24] a significant amount of patients with pSS were found to have low maximal expiratory flow rate, which is often considered a more sensitive measurement of early airflow obstruction, particularly in the small airways. However, clinically relevant airway obstruction was only observed in 10% of the patients.[24] This finding suggests the need to further examine subclinical airway obstruction in pSS. Although a minority displays overt symptomatology, significant airway damage may still occur.

Lymphocytic interstitial pneumonitis (LIP) is one of the most common lung pathologies seen in patients with pSS. LIP is a benign lymphoproliferative disorder characterized by diffuse infiltration of the pulmonary parenchymal interstitum by polyclonal lymphocytes and plasma cells that localize to the interstitial septa often filling the alveolar spaces.[25,26] It commonly favors females and presents at about the sixth decade of life. It presents with nonspecific respiratory symptoms, such as dry cough and dyspnea. On physical examination lung auscultation often reveals bibasilar crackles.[27] These vague symptoms may again delay recognition as an EGM associated with pSS. In one study, the mean time from presentation to diagnosis exceeded 15 months.[28] Rarely, a patient with LIP may also present with fever, night sweats, and weight loss[26] leading to an incorrect diagnosis of infection. Radiographic findings of nonspecific bilateral reticular or reticulonodular opacities may lead to treatment with multiple courses of antibiotics before an inflammatory cause is considered. High-resolution CT scan is the imaging modality of choice and shows a characteristic pattern consisting of areas of ground-glass attenuation with scattered thin-walled cysts in about 50% of patients with LIP.[29,30] It has been reported that 25% of LIP cases may be associated with Sjögren's syndrome.[26] Although a diagnosis of LIP may be attributed to a systemic disease, such as pSS, it is also important to remember that LIP may also be associated with other diseases, such as HIV. LIP may coexist with follicular bronchiolitis and these two entities can progress to lymphoma,[25] an important consideration when managing patients with Sjögren's syndrome.

Nonspecific interstitial pneumonia (NSIP) is also a common form of interstitial lung disease in pSS. It has been reported in up to 61% of pSS patient's lung manifestations. Prevalence is more commonly reported to range between 28% and 33%.[31–33] NSIP presents with cough and dyspnea but is more commonly associated with fever compared with LIP. Pulmonary function testing demonstrates a restrictive pattern with decreased diffusing capacity of lung for carbon monoxide, a pattern commonly seen in pSS. CT demonstrates increased reticular markings, traction bronchiectasis, lobar volume loss, and ground-glass opacities.[34] Histologically, alveolar wall interstitial inflammation is seen and can lead to fibrosis.[25]

A retrospective study performed by Parambil and colleagues[31] examined 18 patients with pSS with suspected interstitial lung disease. All had lung biopsy performed. Although a variety of histopathologic findings were seen including NSIP, LIP, usual interstitial pneumonia (UIP), and organizing pneumonia, UIP tended to have the greatest progression of lung disease despite treatment.[31]

Pulmonary hypertension can be a severe and debilitating disease. Fortunately, it is a rare manifestation of pSS and is far less common in pSS than in other connective tissue diseases, such as scleroderma. The pathogenesis of pulmonary hypertension in pSS remains unclear. Some have proposed that it results from vasculitis with prolonged vasospasm followed by structural vessel remodeling leading to thrombotic obstruction of the pulmonary arterioles.[25] Patients with pSS with pulmonary hypertension may also have Raynaud phenomenon, vasculitis, and interstitial lung disease.[26]

Although the clinical presentation may vary, it is clear that pulmonary manifestations are common EGMs in pSS. Although nonproductive cough often occurs, it is important to remember the variety of ways the lung involvement may impact outcome. In a study of a Norwegian population with Sjögren's syndrome, using the Medical Outcomes Study 36-Item Short Form Health Survey, patients with pSS and pulmonary involvement had greater impaired physical functioning compared with patients with pSS without pulmonary involvement.[35] In the same study there was a fourfold increase in mortality after 10 years of disease in patients with pSS with lung disease compared with patients with pSS without lung disease.[35] Recognizing and treating early manifestations of pulmonary involvement of Sjögren's syndrome may lead to better control of the disease and a better quality of life for the patient.

MUSCULOSKELETAL MANIFESTATIONS

Arthritis and arthralgias are among the most common EGMs seen in Sjögren's syndrome (**Box 4**).

> **Box 4**
> **Musculoskeletal involvement**
>
> - Nonerosive arthritis has been reported in up to 40% of patients with pSS.
> - Arthralgias associated with pSS are reported as more symmetric in distribution, whereas arthritis is more asymmetric.
> - PSS may have a modifying effect on coexisting rheumatoid arthritis because less severe radiographic changes have been noted in the presence of pSS and rheumatoid arthritis compared with rheumatoid arthritis alone.
> - Fibromyalgia syndrome has been reported in up to 20% of patients with pSS. Patients with fibromyalgia syndrome alone have been reported to have a lower pain threshold.

Nonerosive arthritis in patients with pSS has been reported to be 40%.[1] The spectrum of joint pathology in pSS relationship has yet to be fully understood.

In a study of 48 patients with pSS it was observed that 26 (54%) had symptoms or signs of arthralgia or arthritis.[36] In 31% of these, arthralgias were reported as occurring before sicca symptoms developed.[36] The distribution of joint symptoms was found to be mostly symmetric in cases of reported arthralgias but cases of true arthritis had a more asymmetric presentation.[36] Characterization of joint pain was mild to moderate rather than severe using the Ritchie joint pain scale in 95% of the cases.[36]

Secondary Sjögren's syndrome is often defined as the development of the sicca component of Sjögren's syndrome in a patient with a major connective tissue disease, such as RA. Nonetheless, it has been reported that an inflammatory arthropathy consistent with RA can occur months to years after a diagnosis of pSS. Khan and Carsons[37] reported six cases where patients with longstanding pSS developed RA requiring oral or biologic disease-modifying antirheumatic drugs. As reported by Pease and colleagues,[36] patients with diagnoses of both RA and Sjögren's syndrome were found to have less salivary gland enlargement, purpuric vasculitis, leucopenia, and positive antinuclear antibody (ANA) titers compared with patients with Sjögren's syndrome alone. When comparing radiographs between patients with RA alone with those with both Sjögren's syndrome and RA it was observed that patients with RA without Sjögren's syndrome had more advanced radiographic changes.[38] Although additional studies are needed, it is interesting to note that the copresence of Sjögren's syndrome may have a modifying effect on the severity of RA.

The presence of joint pain in a patient with pSS should prompt a thorough musculoskeletal evaluation. Arthralgias and fleeting synovitis seem to be fairly common EGMs associated with pSS. The development of persistent, symmetric synovitis particularly if accompanied by deformity, radiographic erosion, and anti-cyclic citrullinated peptide antibody should raise suspicion for an overlap of pSS and RA. This is important to identify because treatment may need to include oral and biologic disease-modifying antirheumatic drugs (discussed in the article by Wu elsewhere in this issue).

Diffuse musculoskeletal aches and pains may indicate the presence of fibromyalgia syndrome (FMS). FMS has been reported to be present in approximately 20% of patients with pSS.[39,40] Priori and colleagues[40] studied the relationship between fatigue and pSS disease activity and reported that 7 out of 35 patients with pSS also fulfilled criteria for FMS. No differences were found in disease duration, Sjögren's disease damage index, and Sjögren's syndrome disease activity index indicating that FMS can contribute to fatigue in pSS but does not entirely account for it.[40] Ostuni and colleagues[39] studied the clinical difference in patients with pSS and FMS compared with patients with primary FMS and reported no difference in the number of tender points between the two groups but a lower pain threshold in patients with primary FMS. Treatment of FMS in Sjögren's syndrome is discussed in the article by Wu elsewhere in this issue.

VASCULITIS

Among the EGMs reported in Sjögren's syndrome, one of the more significant in terms of outcome is vasculitis (**Box 5**). The prevalence of vasculitis in pSS has been reported to be between 5% and 10%.[41–43] The precise cause of vasculitis in Sjögren's syndrome is not entirely known; however, it is hypothesized that a B cell–driven autoimmune process produces antibodies against SS-A and SS-B antigens that form circulating immune complexes that are not properly cleared.[41,44,45] In addition, there seems to be an immunogenetic basis to SS-A and SS-B production and immune complex clearance efficiency. In an article by Moutsopoulos and colleagues[46] there was an increased frequency of HLA-DRW3 antigen in patients with pSS compared with those with secondary Sjögren's syndrome. This association was found to be restricted to patients with SS-A and/or SS-B antibodies.[47] Salmon and colleagues[48] reported that there seems to be a decrease in phagocytosis of Ig-coated red blood cells by blood monocytes in normal individuals with HLADR2 or DR3, which may contribute to impaired immune complex clearance and a predisposition to vasculitis.

In the early 1980s, Alexander[19] and Provost and colleagues[49] reported a study of 22 patients with pSS with a documented skin rash. After a skin biopsy 19 were found to have cutaneous vasculitis with 14 of them being classified as leukocytoclastic vasculitis. In a larger study looking at 558 patients with pSS, 52 had a form of cutaneous vasculitis. Patients with cutaneous vasculitis had more severe disease and more EGMs than those without.[42] The lower extremities were the most common areas affected by leukocytoclastic vasculitis in pSS.[42]

Systemic vasculitis occurring in pSS has been described in several case reports and involves medium- and small-sized arteries.[50] One study of 70 patients with Sjögren's syndrome found that nine had vasculitis; some had an acute necrotizing arteritis of medium-sized vessels.[51] The entire vascular wall was infiltrated with inflammatory cells and fibrinoid necrosis was present.[51] Acute necrotizing vasculitis in pSS is described as having a similar clinical presentation to polyarteritis nodosa but lacking the typical aneurysmal formation.[51] A more severe course of Sjögren's was associated with acute necrotizing vasculitis compared with the course of Sjögren's seen in other types of vasculitis.[51] Leukocytoclastic vasculitis, a type of vasculitis where the capillaries and venules are infiltrated with polymorphonuclear leukocytes, and lymphocytic vasculitis, where small vessels are surrounded by and occasionally infiltrated by mononuclear cells, predominantly affect the skin and were seen in 44% of the patients biopsied.[51] Endarteritis obliterans, which is characterized as a noninflammatory obstructive

---

Box 5
pSS associated with vasculitis

- The prevalence of vasculitis in pSS has been reported to be between 5% and 10%.

- Of the end organs involved, skin and the peripheral nerves are most commonly involved.

- Patients with pSS and vasculitis may have more severe disease and a greater number of EGMs compared with patients with pSS without vasculitis.

- The development of lymphoproliferative disorders has been associated with palpable purpura, low C4, and mixed cryoglobulinemia.

vasculitis involving the medium-sized vessels, was also seen in 44% and was believed to represent a healed pre-existing vasculitis.[51]

Of the end organs affected by the vasculitides described by Tsokos and colleagues,[51] the skin and peripheral nerves were most consistently involved. Of the patients with Sjögren's and vasculitis, all had accompanying anemia and positive rheumatoid factor.[51] Seven of the nine patients had ANA and low complement.[51] Positive rheumatoid factor, ANA, and cryoglobulins have been reported in patients with pSS and vasculitis in other studies.[41,42] In a study by Skopouli and colleagues[52] of 261 patients with pSS, it was observed that the development of lymphoproliferative disorders was consistently associated with the presence of pupura, low C4, and a mixed monoclonal cryoglobulinemia at the time of diagnosis. During follow-up, low C4 and mixed monoclonal cryoglobulinemia were the most important predictors.

Vasculitis does not seem to be as frequent as some of the other EGMs of pSS. However, vasculitis should be sought when evaluating a patient with pSS because its consequences can be very severe. In the study by Tsokos and colleagues,[51] one patient died from gallbladder perforation secondary to necrotizing vasculitis despite treatment. Vasculitis more commonly can result in neurologic deficit, chronic cutaneous ulcerations, and seems to confer risk for non-Hodgkin lymphoma. Complete evaluation should always be performed when evaluating patients with pSS because although rash is the most common presentation of vasculitis in Sjögren's syndrome, it may not always be present when internal organ involvement occurs.

SUMMARY

Sjögren's syndrome is known as a chronic autoimmune disease that affects the exocrine glands but as reported is well known also to affect extraglandular sites. It is important to be aware of all the ways in which Sjögren's may present. Symptoms thought not typically related to Sjögren's syndrome, such as neuropathic pain or dry cough, may go unrecognized for some time before being attributed to Sjögren's syndrome. The need for thorough evaluation to screen for and promptly identify EGMs with rapid institution of treatment may lead to a better quality of life and decreased morbidity in patients with pSS.

REFERENCES

1. Hernandez-Molina G, Michel-Peregrina M, Bermúdez-Bermejo P, et al. Early and late extraglandular manifestations in primary Sjogren's syndrome. Clin Exp Rheumatol 2012;30(3):455.
2. Mori K, Iijima M, Koike H, et al. The wide spectrum of clinical manifestations in Sjogren's syndrome-associated neuropathy. Brain 2005; 128:2518–34.
3. Manilow K, Yannakakis GD, Glusman SM, et al. Subacute sensory neuronopathy secondary to dorsal root ganglionitis in primary Sjogren's syndrome. Ann Neurol 1986;20:535–7.
4. Griffin JW, Cornblath DR, Alexander E, et al. Ataxic sensory neuropathy and dorsal root ganglionitis associated with Sjogren's syndrome. Ann Neurol 1990;27:304–15.
5. Sghirlanzoni A, Payerson D, Lauria G. Sensory neuron diseases. Lancet Neurol 2005;4:349–61.
6. Dalakas MC. Chronic idiopathic ataxic neuropathy. Ann Neurol 1986;19:545–54.
7. Grant IA, Hunder GC, Homburger HA, et al. Peripheral neuropathy associated with sicca complex. Neurology 1997;48:855–62.
8. Pavlakis P, Alexopoulos H, Kosmidis ML, et al. Peripheral neuropathies in Sjögren's syndrome: a critical update on clinical features and pathogenic mechanisms. J Autoimmun 2012;39:27–33.
9. Segal B, Carpenter A, Walk D. Involvement of nervous system pathways in primary Sjögren's syndrome. Rheum Dis Clin North Am 2008;34:885–906.
10. Alexander GE, Provost TT, Stevens MB, et al. Sjogren's syndrome: central nervous system manifestations. Neurology 1901;31.1091–0.
11. Alexander EL, Manilow K, Lejewski JE, et al. Primary Sjögren's syndrome with central nervous system disease mimicking multiple sclerosis. Ann Intern Med 1986;104:323–30.
12. Noseworthy JH, Bass BH, Vandervoort MK, et al. The prevalence of primary Sjögren's syndrome in a multiple sclerosis population. Ann Neurol 1989; 25(1):95–8.
13. De Seze J, Devos D, Castelnovo G, et al. The prevalence of Sjögren's syndrome in patients with primary progressive multiple sclerosis. Neurology 2001;57(8):1359–63.
14. Vitali C, Bombardieri S, Moutsopoulos HM, et al. Assessment of the European classification criteria for Sjögren's syndrome in a series of clinically defined cases: results of a prospective multicentre study. The European Study Group on Diagnostic Criteria for Sjögren's syndrome. Ann Rheum Dis 1996;55(2):116–21.
15. Coates T, Slavotinek JP, Rischmueller M, et al. Cerebral white matter lesions in primary Sjögren's syndrome: a controlled study. J Rheumatol 1999;26: 1301–5.
16. Tzarouchi L, Tsifetaki N, Konitsiotis S, et al. CNS involvement in primary Sjogren syndrome: assessment of gray and white matter changes with MRI

and voxel-based morphometry. Am J Roentgenol 2011;197(5):1207–12.

17. Alexander EL, Beall SS, Gordon B, et al. Magnetic resonance imaging of cerebral lesions in patients with the Sjogren's syndrome. Ann Intern Med 1988;108:815–23.

18. Govoni M, Bajocchi G, Rizzo N, et al. Neurological involvement in primary Sjogren's syndrome: clinical and instrumental evaluation in a cohort of Italian patients. Clin Rheumatol 1999;18:299–303.

19. Alexander EL. Neurologic disease in Sjogren's syndrome: mononuclear inflammatory vasculopathy affecting central/peripheral nervous system and muscle: a clinical review and update of immunopathogenesis. Rheum Dis Clin North Am 1993;19: 869–908.

20. Valtysodottir ST, Gudbjornsson B, Lindqvist U, et al. Anxiety and depression in patients with primary Sjogren's syndrome. J Rheumatol 2000;27(1):165–9.

21. Strimlan CV, Rosenow EC 3rd, Divertie MB, et al. Pulmonary manifestations of Sjogren's syndrome. Chest 1976;70:354–61.

22. Constantopoulos SH, Papadimitriou CS, Moutsopoulos HM. Respiratory manifestations in primary Sjogren's syndrome. A clinical, functional, and histological study. Chest 1985;88:226–9.

23. Yazisiz V, Arslan G, Ozbudak IH, et al. Lung involvement in patients with primary Sjogren's syndrome: what are the predictors? Ann Rheum Dis 2002;61(6):554–8.

24. Papiris S, Maniati M, Constantopoulos S, et al. Lung involvement in primary Sjogren's syndrome is mainly related to the small airway disease. Ann Rheum Dis 1999;58:61–4.

25. Kokosi M, Riemer E, Highland K. Pulmonary involvement in Sjogren syndrome. Clin Chest Med 2010;31(3):489–500.

26. Dalvi V, Gonzalez E, Lovett L. Lymphocytic interstitial pneumonitis (LIP) in Sjogren's syndrome: a case report and a review of the literature. Clin Rheumatol 2007;26:1339–43.

27. Liebow A, Carrington C. Diffuse pulmonary lymphoreticular infiltrations associated with dysproteinemia. Med Clin North Am 1973;57:809–43.

28. Koss M, Hochholzer L, Langloss J, et al. Lymphoid interstitial pneumonia: clinicopathological and immunopathological findings in 18 cases. Pathology 1987;19:178–85.

29. Johkoh T, Muler NL, Pickford M, et al. Lymphocytic interstitial pneumonia: thin section/CT findings in 22 patients. Radiology 1999;212:567–72.

30. Koyama M, Johkoh T, Honda O, et al. Pulmonary involvement in primary Sjogren's syndrome: spectrum of pulmonary abnormalities and computed tomography findings in 60 patients. J Thorac Imaging 2001;16:94–8.

31. Parambil JG, Myers JL, Lindell RM, et al. Interstitial lung disease in primary Sjogren's syndrome. Chest 2006;130:1489–95.

32. Ito I, Nagai S, Kitaichi M, et al. Pulmonary manifestations of primary Sjogren's syndrome: a clinical, radiologic, and pathologic study. Am J Respir Crit Care Med 2005;171:632–8.

33. Yamadori I, Fujita J, Bandoh S, et al. Nonspecific interstitial pneumonia as pulmonary involvement of primary Sjogren's syndrome. Rheumatol Int 2002;22:89–92.

34. Travis WD, Hunninghake G, King TE Jr, et al. Idiopathic nonspecific interstitial pneumonia: report of an American Thoracic Society project. Am J Respir Crit Care Med 2008;177:1338–47.

35. Palm O, Garen T, Enger TB, et al. Clinical pulmonary involvement in primary Sjogren's syndrome: prevalence, quality of life and mortality. A retrospective study based on registry data. Rheumatology 2013;52:173–9.

36. Pease CT, Shattles W, Barrett NK, et al. The arthropathy of Sjogren's syndrome. Br J Rheumatol 1993;32:609–13.

37. Khan O, Carsons S. Occurrence of rheumatoid arthritis requiring oral and/or biologic diseasemodifying antirheumatic drug therapy following a diagnosis of primary Sjogren's syndrome. J Clin Rheumatol 2012;18(7):356–8.

38. Tsampoulas CG, Skopouli FN, Sartoris DJ, et al. Hand radiographic changes in patients with primary and secondary Sjogren's syndrome. Scand J Rheumatol 1986;15(3):333–9.

39. Ostuni P, Botsios C, Sfriso P, et al. Fibromyalgia in Italian patients with primary Sjogren's syndrome. Joint Bone Spine 2002;69(1):51–7.

40. Priori R, Iannuccelli C, Alessandri C, et al. Fatigue in Sjogren's syndrome: relationship with fibromyalgia, clinical and biologic features. Clin Exp Rheumatol 2010;28(6 Suppl 63):S82–6.

41. Feist E, Hermann KG, Dankof A. Vasculopathy in Sjogren's syndrome. Z Rheumatol 2009;68(4): 305–11 [in German].

42. Ramos-Casals M, Anaya JM, Garcia-Carrasco M, et al. Cutaneous vasculitis in primary Sjogren syndrome: classification and clinical significance of 52 patients. Medicine 2004;83:96–106.

43. Ramos-Casals M, Solans R, Rosas J, et al. GEMESS Study Group: primary Sjogren syndrome in Spain: clinical and immunologic expression in 1010 patients. Medicine 2008;87:210–9.

44. Hamburger MI, Moutsopoulos HM, Lawley TJ, et al. Sjogren's syndrome. A defect in reticuloendothelial system. Fc-receptor-specific clearance. Ann Intern Med 1979;91:534–8.

45. Lawley TJ, Moutsopoulos HM, Katz SI, et al. Demonstration of circulating immune complexes

in Sjogren's syndrome. J Immunol 1979;123:
1382–7.

46. Moutsopoulos HM, Chused TM, Mann DL, et al.
Sjogren's syndrome (sicca syndrome): current issues. Ann Intern Med 1980;92:212–26.

47. Gottenberg JE, Busson M, Loiseau P, et al. In primary Sjogren's syndrome, HLA class 2 is associated exclusively with autoantibody production
and spreading of the autoimmune response.
Arthritis Rheum 2003;48(8):2240–5.

48. Salmon JE, Kimberly RP, Gibofsky A, et al.
Altered phagocytosis by monocytes from HLA-
DR2 and DR3-positive healthy adults is Fc
gamma receptor specific. J Immunol 1986;
136(10):3625–30.

49. Alexander EL, Provost TT. Cutaneous manifestations of primary Sjogren's syndrome: a reflection
of vasculitis and association with anti-Ro (SSA) antibodies. The Journal of Investigative Dermatology
1983;80(5):386–91.

50. Scofield RH. Vasculitis in Sjogren's syndrome. Curr
Rheumatol Rep 2011;13:482–8.

51. Tsokos M, Lazarou SA, Moutsopoulos HM. Vasculitis in primary Sjogren's syndrome. Histologic classification and clinical presentation. Am J Clin
Pathol 1987;88(1):26–31.

52. Skopouli F, Dafni U, Ioannidis J, et al. Clinical evo-
lution, and morbidity and mortality of primary Sjogren's syndrome. Semin Arthritis Rheum 2000;29(5):
296–304.

Management of Extraglandular Manifestations of Primary Sjögren's Syndrome

Jason J. Wu, DO[a,b], Steven E. Carsons, MD[a,c],*

KEYWORDS

- Sjögren's syndrome • Joint pain • NSAIDs • Anti-TNF

KEY POINTS

- Primary Sjögren's syndrome can have multiple extra-glandular manifestations ranging from mild to severe.
- Treatment for extra-glandular manifestations is organ specific and therapies are targeted based on the primary organs involved.
- Preferred treatment options used for extra-glandular manifestations of Sjögren's syndrome are usually extrapolated from the physician's experience in treating similar manifestations in other auto-immune conditions such as rheumatoid arthritis and systemic lupus erythematous.
- The lack of immunomodulating disease modifying drugs in Sjögren's syndrome can be frustrating for patients dealing with extra-glandular manifestations, however recent advances in the field has made the future look promising for new therapeutic options.

Primary Sjögren's syndrome (pSS) is an autoimmune inflammatory disorder mainly affecting the exocrine glands. Like many autoimmune disorders, however, pSS is a systemic disease in which many different organs may be affected (**Table 1** and article by Ienopolli and Carsons elsewhere in this issue). Sometimes, extraglandular manifestations like purpura, polyneuropathy, and arthritis can be presenting signs of the disease.[1] In other cases, extraglandular involvement may not be as evident and present subclinically in pSS. In evaluating patients with pSS, extraglandular manifestations should be questioned and considered.

Given the large spectrum of clinical manifestations of pSS, ranging from a limited involvement of exocrine glands to widespread systemic features, clinicians have now distinguished 2 variants of the syndrome: an exocrine gland-localized disease, and a systemic syndrome.[2] Although symptomatic therapy may be enough for most patients

with localized glandular symptoms, the lack of immunomodulating disease-modifying drugs in pSS has an important impact on patients with systemic manifestations and severe organ involvement. During the past few years, promising results have been seen with some of the new biologic therapies and others could be considered hypothetically useful in the future for treating extraglandular manifestations of this disorder.

In this article, the current conservative and medical therapies for the more common extraglandular manifestations seen in pSS are reviewed. In addition to reviewing accepted current therapies in pSS, recent research on treatments that are promising for the future are examined as well.

MUSCULOSKELETAL MANIFESTATIONS

Musculoskeletal manifestations, such as arthralgias, myalgias, and nonerosive polyarthritis

a Division of Rheumatology, Allergy and Immunology, Department of Medicine, Winthrop University Hospital, Mineola, NY 11501, USA; b Nassau University Medical Center, East Meadow, NY 11554, USA; c Stony Brook University School of Medicine, Stony Brook, NY 11794, USA
* Corresponding author. Division of Rheumatology, Allergy and Immunology, Department of Medicine, Winthrop University Hospital, Mineola, NY 11501.
E-mail address: scarsons@winthrop.org

Oral Maxillofacial Surg Clin N Am 26 (2014) 101–109
http://dx.doi.org/10.1016/j.coms.2013.09.009
1042-3699/14/$ – see front matter © 2014 Elsevier Inc. All rights reserved.

Table 1
Extraglandular manifestations of Sjögren's syndrome

Organ System	Manifestation
Skin	• Xerostosis • Cutaneous vasculitis • Other skin lesions (erythema nodosum, livedo reticulares, lichen planus, vitiligo)
Joints/muscles	• Arthralgia/arthritis • Myalgia/myopathy
Pulmonary	• Interstitial lung disease • Pulmonary fibrosis • Pulmonary hypertension • Small airway obstruction • Bronchiectasis
Cardiovascular/ circulatory	• Pericarditis • Arrythmia • Raynaud phenomenon
Nervous system	• Peripheral neuropathy • Cranial neuropathy • Central nervous system involvement • Autonomic neuropathy
Gastrointestinal	• Dysphagia • Esophageal dysmotility • Autoimmune hepatitis • Pancreatitis
Urogenital	• Interstitial nephritis with renal tubular acidosis • Interstitial cystitis

Modified from Vissink A, Bootsma H, Spijkervet F, et al. Current and future challenges in primary Sjogren's syndrome. Curr Pharm Biotechnol 2012;13:2026–45.

affecting mainly the small joints, are one of the most common comorbidities in pSS and may be difficult to manage. It is important to determine if the cause of pain is more articular or muscular in nature. If arthralgias or polyarthritis is the dominant manifesting symptom, agents used to treat articular manifestations of other connective tissue disease conditions like rheumatoid arthritis (RA) or systemic lupus erythematosus (SLE) should be efficacious. However, fibromyalgia is a common coexisting condition in pSS and treatments effective for fibromyalgia are more appropriate for noninflammatory muscular symptoms in pSS. It is also important to differentiate between tenderness secondary to parotid or other glandular inflammation versus arthritic involvement of the temporomandibular joint in pSS. It may be difficult sometimes to differentiate between parotid and temporomandibular joint involvement, but therapies between glandular inflammation and

arthritic conditions can differ greatly, thus further demonstrating the importance of determining cause of pain in pSS.

Initially, nonsteroidal anti-inflammatory drugs (NSAIDs) or analgesics are the commonly applied treatment of musculoskeletal symptoms in pSS.[2] There are many NSAIDs from which to choose. Although the efficacy of various NSAIDs is similar, an individual's response to therapy can be highly variable.[3] Acetaminophen may have the best safety profile, but its analgesic effect is mild.

Stronger analgesics like opioid (narcotic) therapy have been used in pSS. Opioid therapy in the treatment of more severe forms of acute pain is well established, but opioid administration in chronic pain remains controversial given their addiction potential. The decision to begin long-term opioid therapy in pSS must be weighed carefully.

If a patient's musculoskeletal complaints are more articular and determined to be inflammatory in cause, preferred therapy is based on experience from similar rheumatologic conditions such as RA and SLE. The efficacy of hydroxychloroquine and methotrexate in RA and SLE subsequently led to these medications being studied in pSS. Primary Sjögren's patients with articular symptoms showed improvement when taking hydroxychloroquine over a 1- to 2-year period compared with baseline.[4–6] However, additional randomized controlled trials must be done with hydroxychloroquine. Methotrexate also fared well for arthritis in 1-year studies compared with baseline.[4,7] Again, none of the studies were controlled studies. Although not primarily given for musculoskeletal symptoms in pSS, a few case reports have shown Rituximab to improve articular symptoms when given to several pSS patients.[8] Low-dose corticosteroids are sometimes used and may be needed to control persistent symptoms in pSS.[2] Anti-tumor necrosis factor (TNF) agents such as etanercept, adalimumab, and infliximab have taken center stage for the treatment of autoimmune-rheumatic diseases in the last decade. However, unlike the success found in modulating RA, they were found to have a lack of efficacy for sicca (dry eyes and dry mouth) symptoms in pSS.[1,9] Although ineffective for sicca, anti-TNF agents could be considered for inflammatory polyarthritis refractory to other agents. On the other hand, questions regarding lymphoma risk in anti-TNF agents temper enthusiasm for these agents in pSS.

Recent interest has emphasized nutrition and inflammatory arthritis. Supplements, particularly omega-3 fatty acids and vitamin D, have been studied in the past decade for SLE, RA, and other connective tissue diseases. Omega-3 fatty acids may have a benefit for sicca symptoms,[10] but no studies have shown a benefit for extraglandular symptoms in pSS. Many of the studies involving omega-3 fatty acids and inflammatory arthritis have been inconclusive, but some have shown that in high doses (at least >2 g/day), omega-3 fatty acids can have an anti-inflammatory effect and reduce frequency of NSAID use.[11,12] Vitamin D deficiency has been linked to diffuse musculoskeletal complaints and risk of vitamin D deficiency is increased in autoimmune conditions such as SLE, RA, pSS, and scleroderma.[13,14] Although vitamin D supplementation is good practice for the prevention of osteoporosis in autoimmune conditions, we are not aware of any good, randomized trials that have shown a reduction in muscle complaints with repletion of vitamin D.

Muscular symptoms in pSS may resemble those seen with fibromyalgia; therefore, use of US Food and Drug Administration (FDA) approved medications for fibromyalgia are an option. There are currently 3 FDA medications approved for fibromyalgia: pregabalin, duloxetine, and milnacipran. Duloxetine and milnacipran are antidepressants that have been efficacious in chronic pain syndromes. Although not FDA approved for fibromyalgia, other selective serotonin reuptake inhibitors and tricyclic antidepressants have been used with success in myalgias in pSS. Pregabalin and other anticonvulsants are effective for chronic pain therapy, particularly for neuropathic pain with reasonable results. Mechanisms of action for the anticonvulsants are different and not fully understood. These medications used for chronic pain syndromes can be drying and are best used at low doses. Other choices that may be better tolerated include trazodone, venlafaxine, tizanidine, and zaleplon.[3]

FATIGUE

Fatigue is a common complaint and can be associated with a wide range of chronic diseases. Even in healthy adults, 11% to 20% report persistent fatigue.[15] In patients with autoimmune diseases, prevalence of fatigue is much higher and can reach 60% to 70%. In pSS, fatigue is reported by patients as worsening their overall quality of life. The problem with treating fatigue in pSS is that it is difficult to demonstrate an association between fatigue severity and other measures of Sjögren's disease activity (eg, sicca, serologies, extraglandular manifestations).

The initial approach to this complex problem begins with a thorough history and physical examination to characterize the fatigue. Medication lists should be reviewed and patients should be screened for anemia, thyroid disease, and depression. In addition, sleep studies to rule out sleep disorders can be considered. Obstructive sleep apnea has been found to be increased in pSS and may be a useful target to improve quality of life.[16] Once treatable medical causes of fatigue are ruled out, conservative treatment measures may be used to relieve fatigue in pSS. These methods include counseling the patient on proper sleep hygiene (**Box 1**).

For pSS patients, nocturnal glandular dryness may disturb sleep and a room humidifier can be helpful. Other conservative recommendations include encouraging ocular lubricants (Refresh PM) or gels (GenTeal gel) instead of using artificial tears for longer lasting relief. Bedtime doses of oral secretagogues (pilocarpine or cevimeline) are useful. Finally, the mouth may be coated with moisturizing gels (Oral Balance, Orajel) to alleviate nighttime symptoms.[17]

Some physicians hypothesize that fatigue in pSS is mediated by the systemic inflammatory response that characterizes the disease. If fatigue is preventing the patient from carrying out daily activities, it is reasonable to undertake a treatment trial with immunosuppressive drugs that can decrease systemic inflammation and possibly alleviate fatigue. Hydroxychloroquine seems to have the most positive data in alleviating fatigue.[6,18] Given rituximab's positive results in treating other symptoms of pSS, there is potential in this medication. Studies have suggested that treatment with rituximab may alleviate fatigue,[19,20] but these

---

Box 1
Tips to achieve restful sleep

- Keep a regular sleep schedule for going to bed and getting up
- Avoid taking daytime naps
- Try to get at least 8.5 hours of sleep per night, or longer if you wake up a lot
- Do not use caffeine within 6 hours of bedtime
- Try to exercise regularly for at least 20 minutes a day, but do not exercise right before bed
- Create a dark, cool, quiet, and secure environment for sleep
- Do not go to bed hungry
- Do not work or watch TV in the bedroom
- Try a warm bath before bedtime to relax aching muscles and relieve stress

Adapted from Mishra R, Vivino F. Diagnosis and management of fatigue. In: Wallace D, editor. The Sjogren's book. 4th edition. New York: Oxford; 2012. p. 228–34. Chapter 23.

studies must be reproduced on a larger scale. Also, the long-term benefit of rituximab in pSS has not been evaluated. Other immunomodulators studied include azathioprine and IL-1 Inhibitors, but these trials had a small sample size and short treatment duration.[21,22]

Fibromyalgia can be a concomitant disorder in primary pSS patients and can complicate the assessment of fatigue. Treatment of fibromyalgia with current FDA-approved medications, pregabalin, duloxetine, and milnacipran, may be beneficial. However, as stated earlier, these medications can be drying and may worsen the patient's overall disease.[3]

Recently, the endogenous steroid hormone supplement, dehydroepiandrosterone, has drawn interest in treatment of autoimmune diseases such as SLE and pSS. Two studies have not shown a superior effect for dehydroepiandrosterone over placebo in pSS.[23,24]

NEUROLOGIC MANIFESTATIONS

The treatment of neurologic manifestations is confounded by the wide variety of nervous system manifestations that are reported in pSS. Neurologic manifestations can consist of central nervous system (CNS) disease, cranial neuropathies, and peripheral nerve disease. Within the spectrum of peripheral nerve manifestations are small- and large-fiber neuropathies, sensory ataxic neuropathy, mononeuritis multiplex, and autonomic neuropathy (see article discussing Neurologic Manifestations by Ienopolli and Carsons elsewhere in this issue). There are few controlled studies in pSS to provide guidelines for treatment of neurologic manifestations. At present most treatment decisions are based on the clinical scenario, anecdotal reports, physician's experience, and the knowledge of the patient's other medical problems. In addition, the experience in treating other disease (eg, CNS lupus, diabetic neuropathy) provides a rationale for choice of therapy in pSS.[25]

Peripheral neurologic involvement is by far more common than CNS involvement.[2] Small-fiber neuropathy is a painful peripheral polyneuropathy that may be the most common peripheral nervous system manifestation of pSS. Treatment of small-fiber neuropathy is mainly symptomatic and based on neuropsychotropic drugs and conventional analgesics, which can include gabapentin or pregabalin as well as tricyclic antidepressants. Corticosteroids and immunosuppressive drugs are usually unsuccessful in small-fiber neuropathy.[26] Small studies have shown that intravenous immunoglobulin (IVIG) therapy decreased pain in Sjögren's syndrome-associated neuropathy.[27,28]

However, other studies have reported minimal to no improvement with IVIG.[29] Even high doses of corticosteroids have been of little use in Sjögren's associated neuropathy, which is contrary to results seen with peripheral nervous system manifestations of systemic vasculitis. One theory is thought to be that vasculitic neuropathy deficits are severe and dramatic, leading to prompt diagnosis and earlier treatment. In contrast, the clinical course in Sjögren's neuropathy is usually subclinical, often leading to delay in diagnosis. There may only be a tiny therapeutic window before there is destruction and irreversible disability.[25]

Cranial mononeuropathies or polyneuropathies have been reported in pSS. Trigeminal neuropathy is well known to be associated with pSS and is usually indolently progressive, can be bilateral, and generally requires symptomatic treatment. The neuropsychotropic treatments mentioned above have been used in cranial neuropathies as well as antiepileptics such as carbamazepine.[25,30]

Rituximab is a treatment that has been recently proposed for pSS. Case reports have shown benefit of rituximab[26,31] in pSS patients with demyelinating neuropathy, mononeuritis multiplex, and small-fiber neuropathy that were refractory to immunomodulatory therapy such as corticosteroids and IVIG. One recent study from France demonstrated that rituximab was effective in cryoglobulinemia or vasculitis-related peripheral nervous system involvement in pSS, but did not improve symptoms of neurologic involvement without cryoglobulinemia or vasculitis in pSS.[32] The studies with rituximab in pSS are promising, but all had a small population size. Therefore, more studies need to be done to truly assess the efficacy of rituximab in peripheral neuropathy.

Orthostasis due to autonomic neuropathy can cause severe disabling complications and syncope. Initial measures include supportive treatments such as plasma fluid expanders (fludricortisone), and α-adrenergic agonists (midodrine), body stockings, and liberal salt intake.[25] There are no standard guidelines for management of autoimmune-mediated autonomic neuropathy, but if orthostasis is still symptomatic, case reports have shown benefit with IVIG and one case report reported benefit with the anti-TNF agent, Etanercept.[33]

CNS disease is a serious but uncommon problem in pSS. It is not as clearly defined as the peripheral nervous system disease in Sjögren's. CNS involvement in pSS is associated with demyelinating diseases (such as multiple sclerosis, neuromyelitis optica, and transverse myelitis) or a CNS vasculitis with white matter abnormalities.[34] In fact, the differential diagnosis of multiple sclerosis and CNS involvement of pSS can be difficult because their clinical presentations are very similar. Almost all symptoms found in patients with CNS Sjögren's involvement could be attributed to the concomitant presence of multiple sclerosis.[35] CNS disease in pSS usually responds to high-dose corticosteroid therapy. Patients with active and/or progressive disease that are refractory to corticosteroids may need immunomodulating therapy, such as azathioprine, cyclophosphamide, IVIG, or rituximab.[25,34]

CUTANEOUS MANIFESTATIONS

Cutaneous features in pSS may range from mild to severe. The most common skin complaint is xerosis (dry skin). Lymphocytic infiltrates are sometimes seen on skin biopsy around the various structures in the dermis, including hair follicles, oil glands, and eccrine (sweat) glands. Once destroyed, these oil and sweat glands cannot be restored. Treatment of dry skin in pSS is similar to treatment of other causes of dry skin (**Box 2**). The SSA/Ro antibody associated with pSS is also associated with subacute cutaneous lupus, which presents with a widespread skin rash usually in sun-exposed areas. The rash is often responsive to topical or systemic steroids. If more aggressive therapies are needed for chronic or recurrent rashes, hydroxychloroquine is often beneficial. Other therapies include dapsone, methotrexate, and azathioprine.[36]

Cutaneous vasculitis can also occur in pSS and can be localized or accompanied with other systemic features. Vasculitis can involve small- and medium-sized arteries of various organs. When there is a systemic vasculitis in pSS, it is usually associated with cryoglobulinemia.[37] After lymphoma, systemic vasculitis is considered the main autoimmune cause of death in this disease.[2]

When vasculitis is present, infectious causes must be ruled out such as endocarditis and hepatitis, and particularly Hepatitis C, which can be a mimic of pSS. The mainstay of therapy for systemic vasculitis secondary to an autoimmune condition is high-dose corticosteroids and cyclophosphamide. This regimen has been used successfully in systemic vasculitis associated with pSS.[2,38] Once initial treatment with cyclophosphamide is completed, azathioprine may be used for maintenance therapy and to allow tapering of corticosteroids. In refractory cases, plasmapheresis and IVIG are alternative treatments.[39]

Rituximab has been recently FDA approved in the United States for anti-neutrophilic cytoplasmic antibodies (ANCA) associated vasculitis and has now been studied and used off-label for other causes of systemic vasculitis including

---

> **Box 2**
> **Tips for dealing with dry skin**
>
> - Take short, lukewarm showers. Lukewarm water does not remove skin oils as completely as hot water.
> - Use gentle bath bars or the low-/no-residue glycerin bars, no harsh deodorant soaps.
> - After bathing, pat dry and moisturize.
> - Moisturize frequently with one of the following techniques:
>   - Trap moisture in the skin, immediately after bathing or showering. While the skin is still damp or moist, apply a thin layer of petrolatum or bath oil.
>   - Drag moisture in the skin with products that contain chemicals such as urea, glycerin, lactic, or similar metabolic or α-hydroxy acids.
>   - Repair the skin's protective barrier function and thereby retain or trap the skin's natural moisture. These products are based on naturally occurring chemicals called ceramides (CeraVe, Aveeno Eczema Care).
> - Avoid fabric softeners, whether in the washer or in the dryer. They may irritate or dry the skin. Use laundry detergents that are free from dyes, fragrances, and preservatives.
> - Drink plenty of water and remain well hydrated.
> - Use a humidifier.
> - Swimming is permissible but may also irritate or dry the skin. Patients should shower after swimming and then immediately use a moisturizer.
>
> *Adapted from* Ray T, Fenyk J Jr. Treatment of other sicca symptoms: dry skin. In: Wallace D, editor. The Sjögren's book. 4th edition. New York: Oxford; 2012. p. 222–3. Chapter 22B.

cryoglobulinemic vasculitis. It would be logical to study Rituximab's efficacy in systemic vasculitis associated with pSS. As mentioned earlier, rituximab was found to be efficacious in cryoglobulinemia or vasculitis-related peripheral nervous system involvement in pSS,[32] but, as of this publication, the authors are not aware of any study showing Rituximab's efficacy on only cutaneous vasculitis associated with pSS.

OTHER MAJOR ORGAN SYSTEM INVOLVEMENT

Other major organ systems that can be affected by pSS include cardiac (pericarditis, arrhythmias), pulmonary (interstitial lung disease, pulmonary fibrosis, pulmonary hypertension), and renal (interstitial nephritis, renal tubular acidosis).[40–42] Managing organ involvement in pSS includes treatment of the primary organ involved (eg, mucolytics for pulmonary disease or electrolyte and base replacement for renal manifestations). For severe organ manifestations, immunomodulating disease-modifying agents used to attenuate the inflammatory process of Sjögren's may be of benefit. This list of agents has been discussed in this article and includes hydroxychloroquine, azathioprine, rituximab, and methotrexate. These agents usually work systemically and can have beneficial effects on more than one area of involvement at a time.[40]

FUTURE DIRECTIONS

So far, some of the more common systemic therapies targeted for the more common

Table 2
Summary of oral immunomodulating and biologic agents used in extraglandular manifestations of Sjögren's syndrome

Agent	Possible Benefit in Extraglandular Symptoms of Sjögren's	Common Adverse Effects	Other Comments
Methotrexate	• Inflammatory arthritis	• GI intolerance • Elevated LFTs, recommend checking LFTs every 4–8 wk • Pulmonary toxicity, recommend checking radiograph at baseline • Alopecia • Pregnancy category X	Give with folic acid or leucovorin to decrease risk of marrow suppression
Hydroxychloroquine	• Fatigue • Inflammatory arthritis • Rash	• Hyperpigmentation • Retinopathy, rare	Ophthalmologic examinations at baseline, then recommend every 6–12 mo
Rituximab	• Inflammatory arthritis • Vasculitis • Demyelinating neuropathy • Mononeuritis multiplex	• Infusion reaction • Immune suppression • Hepatitis reactivation • Possible progressive multifocal leukoencephalopathy, rare • GI obstruction or perforation • Cardiotoxicity	Recommend screening for Hepatitis B before infusion
Anti-TNF agents	• Inflammatory arthritis	• Infusion or injection site reaction • Immune suppression • Hepatitis reactivation • Tuberculosis reactivation • Possible lymphoma risk • CHF • Drug-induced lupus	Recommend tuberculosis and hepatitis screening at baseline, caution in Sjögren's syndrome given lymphoma risk
Belimumab	• Inflammatory arthritis • Rash • Fatigue	• Infusion reaction • Possible immune suppression • Insomnia/anxiety	
Abatacept	• Inflammatory arthritis	• Infusion or injection site reaction • Immune suppression • Hypertension	Recommend hepatitis and tuberculosis screening at baseline

extra-glandular manifestations of pSS have been discussed. There are many other agents that have piqued interest in glandular symptoms of pSS that may work on extraglandular manifestations as well. These medications, especially those that suppress B-lymphocytes, are under active investigation because there is abundant evidence that B cells are a major pathogenic factor in pSS.[9]

Rituximab

Rituximab, a chimeric humanized monoclonal antibody specific for the B-cell surface molecule CD-20, has already been discussed in this article in sections on musculoskeletal, neurologic, and cutaneous manifestations. It is of note that some rheumatologists are using this medication off label in patients with pSS for symptoms that are refractory to conventional therapies.

Epratuzumab

Epratuzumab is a fully humanized monoclonal antibody specific for the B-cell surface molecule CD-22. This medication is similar to Rituximab in that it inhibits specific B-cell antigens. However, this molecule is newer and there is much less experience with this therapy. In a phase I/II trial, Epratuzumab was effective not only in glandular manifestations of pSS but also for subjective symptom scores for fatigue.[43] Interestingly, there seemed to be more responders at 6 months than at 6 weeks. Other extraglandular manifestations were not studied in this trial.

Belimumab

Belimumab is a human antibody that is a B-cell activating factor antagonist that has recently received FDA approval in SLE. Belimumab seems to work best for non-major organ involvement SLE. It has some efficacy in articular, cutaneous, and fatigue symptoms in SLE.[1] No study to the authors' knowledge has examined belimumab and pSS but, given the efficacy in SLE, this may be another target for therapy in pSS.

Abatacept

Abatacept is more known for T-cell inhibition because it is a fully human soluble costimulation modulator that selectively targets the CD80/CD86:CD28 costimulatory signal required for full T-cell activation. However, this molecule also inhibits the T-cell-dependent activation of B cells. Abatacept seems to be safe and effective in RA[44] and is currently FDA approved for RA patients usually those refractory to anti-TNF therapy. Currently, abatacept has not been tested in pSS,

but it could be a good alternative to B-cell depletion therapy in pSS.[1] In addition, abatacept's efficacy on inflammatory arthritis in RA may make it a good treatment option for inflammatory articular manifestations of pSS because anti-TNF agents have an increased risk for lymphoma.

SUMMARY

Although many pSS patients have limited glandular disease that can be controlled with conservative measures, certain patients may have various extraglandular manifestations that can be severe and have a substantial impact on patients' quality of life and their daily activities. For these patients, the lack of immunomodulating disease-modifying drugs in pSS can be frustrating. This article reviewed therapies of interest currently being used or studied in the treatment of extraglandular manifestations of pSS including conservative, medical, and alternative treatments. Some common conservative therapies and mild medications that may help in extra-glandular symptoms were reviewed (Table 2). For severe, systemic manifestations, however, it was found that many current treatments have only been studied in small samples in pSS. Therefore, more randomized, controlled clinical trials using larger populations must be done before efficacy is truly determined. Although frustrating for patients and physicians dealing and treating severe extraglandular manifestations of pSS, respectively, the future is brighter than it ever has been for pSS therapy with continued innovative clinical development efforts in pSS research.

REFERENCES

1. Vissink A, Bootsma H, Spijkervet F, et al. Current and future challenges in primary Sjogren's syndrome. Curr Pharm Biotechnol 2012;13:2026–45.

2. Vitale C, Palombi G, Cataleta P. Treating Sjogren's syndrome: insights for the clinician. Ther Adv Musculoskelet Dis 2010;2:155–66.

3. Chen L. Management of chronic musculoskeletal pain. In: Wallace D, editor. The Sjogren's book. 4th edition. New York: Oxford; 2012. p. 235–40 Chapter 24.

4. Fauchais A, Ouattara B, Gondran G, et al. Articular manifestations in primary Sjogren's syndrome: clinical significance and prognosis of 188 patients. Rheumatology 2010;49:1164–72.

5. Fox R, Dixon R, Guarrasi V, et al. Treatment of primary Sjogren's syndrome with hydroxchloroquine: a retrospective open-label study. Lupus 1996; 5(Suppl 1):S31–6.

6. Kruize A, Hene R, Kallenberg C, et al. Hydroxychloroquine treatment for primary Sjogren's syndrome: a two

year double blind crossover trial. Ann Rheum Dis 1993;52:360–4.

7. Skopouli FN, Jagiello P, Tsifetaki N, et al. Methotrexate in primary Sjogren's syndrome. Clin Exp Rheumatol 1996;14(5):555–8.

8. Covelli M, Lanciano E, Tartaglia P, et al. Rituximab treatment for Sjogren syndrome-associated non-Hodgkin's lymphoma: case series. Rheumatol Int 2012;32:3281–4.

9. Peri Y, Agmon-Levin N, Theodor E, et al. Sjogren's syndrome, the old and the new. Best Pract Res Clin Rheumatol 2012;26:105–17.

10. Miljanovic B, Trivedi K, Dana M, et al. Relation between dietary n-3 and n-6 fatty acids and clinically diagnosed dry eye syndrome in women. Am J Clin Nutr 2005;82:887–93.

11. Lee Y, Bae S, Song G. Omega-3 polyunsaturated fatty acids and the treatment of rheumatoid arthritis: a meta-analysis. Arch Med Res 2012;45:356–62.

12. Calder P. Omega-3 polyunsaturated fatty acids and inflammatory processes: nutrition or pharmacology? Br J Clin Pharmacol 2013;75:645–62.

13. Wilson J. Vitamin D and Sjogren's syndrome. In: Wallace D, editor. The Sjogren's book. 4th edition. New York: Oxford; 2012. p. 271–5 Chapter 28.

14. Kostoglou-Athanassiou I, Athanassiou P, Lyraki A, et al. Vitamin D and rheumatoid arthritis. Ther Adv Endocrinol Metab 2012;3:181–7.

15. Priori R, Iannuccelli C, Alessandri C, et al. Fatigue in Sjogren's syndrome: relationship with fibromyalgia, clinical and biological features. Clin Exp Rheumatol 2010;28:S82–6.

16. Usmani ZA, Hlavac M, Rischmueller M, et al. Sleep disordered breathing in patients with primary Sjögren's syndrome: a group controlled study. Sleep Med 2012;13:1066–70.

17. Mishra R, Vivino F. Diagnosis and management of fatigue. In: Wallace D, editor. The Sjogren's book. 4th edition. New York: Oxford; 2012. p. 228–34 Chapter 23.

18. Venables PJ. Management of patients presenting with Sjogren's syndrome. Best Pract Res Clin Rheumatol 2006;20:791–807.

19. Dass S, Bowman S, Vital E, et al. Reduction of fatigue in Sjogren's syndrome with rituximab: results of a randomised, double-blind, placebo-controlled pilot study. Ann Rheum Dis 2008;67:1541–4.

20. Meijer J, Meiners P, Vissink A, et al. Effectiveness of rituximab treatment in primary Sjogren's syndrome: a randomised, double-blind, palcebo-controlled trial. Arthritis Rheum 2010;62:960–8.

21. Price E, Rigby S, Clancy U, et al. A double blind placebo controlled trial of azathioprine in the treatment of primary Sjogren's syndrome. J Rheumatol 1998; 25:896–9.

22. Norheim K, Harboe E, Goransson L, et al. Interleukin-1 inhibition and fatigue in primary Sjogren's syndrome-a

double blind, randomised clinical trial. PLoS One 2012;7:e30123.

23. Hartkamp A, Geenen R, Godaert G, et al. Effect of dehydroepiandrosterone administration on fatigue, well-being, and functioning in women with primary Sjogren syndrome: a randomised controlled trial. Ann Rheum Dis 2008;67:91–7.

24. Virkki L, Porola P, Forsblad-d'Elia H, et al. Dehydroepiandrosterone (DHEA) substitution treatment for severe fatigue in DHEA-deficient patients with primary Sjogren's syndrome. Arthritis Care Res (Hoboken) 2010;62:118–24.

25. Mandel S, Lopinto-Khoury C, Manon-Espaillat R, et al. Evaluation and management of the neurological manifestations of Sjogren's syndrome. In: Wallace D, editor. The Sjogren's book. 4th edition. New York: Oxford; 2012. p. 249–59 Chapter 26.

26. Sene D, Authier F, Amoura Z, et al. Small fibre neuropathy: diagnostic approach and therapeutic issues, and its association with primary Sjogren's syndrome. Rev Med Interne 2010;31:677–84.

27. Morozumi S, Kawagashira Y, Iijima M, et al. Intravenous immunoglobulin treatment for painful sensory neuropathy associated with Sjogren's syndrome. J Neurol Sci 2009;279:57–61.

28. Rist S, Sellam J, Hachulla E, et al. Experience of intravenous immunoglobulin therapy in neuropathy associated with primary Sjogren's syndrome: a national multicentric retrospective study. Arthritis Care Res 2011;63:1339–44.

29. Mellgren SI, Goransson LG, Omdal R. Primary Sjogren's syndrome associated neuropathy. Can J Neurol Sci 2007;4:280–7.

30. Birnbaum J. Peripheral nervous system manifestations of Sjogren syndrome. Neurologist 2010;16: 287–97.

31. Botez S, Herrmann D. Prolonged remission of a demyelinating neuropathy in a patient with lymphoma and Sjogren's syndrome after rituximab therapy. J Clin Neuromuscul Dis 2010;11:127–31.

32. Mekinian A, Ravaud P, Hatron P, et al. Efficacy of rituximab in primary Sjogren's syndrome with peripheral nervous system involvement: results from the AIR registry. Ann Rheum Dis 2012;71:84–7.

33. Bourcier M, Vinik A. A 41-year-old man with polyarthritis and severe autonomic neuropathy. Ther Clin Risk Manag 2008;4:837–42.

34. Akasbi M, Berenguer J, Saiz A, et al. White matter abnormalities in primary Sjögren syndrome. QJM 2012;105:433–43.

35. Pizova N. The Sjögren's syndrome and multiple sclerosis: similarity and differences. Zh Nevrol Psikhiatr Im S S Korsakova 2012;112:69–74.

36. Ray T, Fenyk J Jr. Treatment of other sicca symptoms: dry skin. In: Wallace D, editor. The Sjogren's book. 4th edition. New York: Oxford; 2012. p. 222–3 Chapter 22B.

37. Ramos-Casals M, Anaya J, Garcia-Carrasco M, et al. Cutaneous vasculitis in primary Sjogren syndrome: classifications and clinical significance of 52 patients. Medicine (Baltimore) 2004;83: 96–106.

38. Souza S, Kuruma K, Andrade D, et al. Primary Sjogren's syndrome with cutaneous vasculitis manifested as leg ulcerations. Rev Bras Reumatol 2004;44: 175–8.

39. Durez P, Tourne L, Feremans W, et al. Dramatic response to intravenous high dose gamma-globulin in refractory vasculitis of the skin associated with Sjogren's syndrome. J Rheumatol 1998;25: 1032–3.

40. Small D. Management of serious internal organ manifestations. In: Wallace D, editor. The Sjogren's book. 4th edition. New York: Oxford; 2012. p. 241–8 Chapter 25.

41. Palm O, Garen T, Berge Enger T, et al. Clincial pulmonary involvement in primary Sjogren's syndrome: prevalence, quality of life and mortality – a retrospective study based on registry data. Rheumatology 2013;52:173–9.

42. Maripuri S, Grande J, Osborn T, et al. Renal involvement in primary Sjogren's syndrome: a clinicopathologic study. Clin J Am Soc Nephrol 2009;4:1423–31.

43. Steinfeld S, Tant L, Burmester G, et al. Epratuzumab (humanised anti-CD22 antibody) in primary Sjögren's syndrome: an open-label phase I/II study. Arthritis Res Ther 2006;8:R129.

44. Genovese M, Schiff M, Luggen M, et al. Efficacy and safety of the selective co-stimulation modulator abatacept following 2 years of treatment in patientswith rheumatoid arthritis and an inadequate response to anti-tumour necrosis factor therapy. Ann Rheum Dis 2008;67:547–54.

Coping Strategies and Support Networks for Sjögren's Syndrome Patients

Andrea Herman, RDH, BS[a],*, Steven Taylor, MBA, BA[b],
Jenene Noll, RN, BSN[c]

KEYWORDS

- Sjögren's syndrome • Coping strategies • Chronic disorder • Autoimmune condition
- Support groups

KEY POINTS

- Although Sjögren's syndrome is a chronic disorder, patients can learn to understand the diagnosis and treat the symptoms by using various coping strategies.
- Sjögren's syndrome patients can join support groups to educate themselves and others about the autoimmune condition and how it affects their body and lifestyle. Many feel that they are alone with this disease, so having a support group helps them understand that this condition affects a great number of others.
- The Sjögren's Syndrome Foundation (SSF) is an important source of credible and valuable information for patients and family members concerned with the condition.

INTRODUCTION

Sjögren's syndrome is a chronic systemic autoimmune inflammatory disorder that is often diagnosed in women in their 40s; however, it can affect all ages as well as men. The three most common symptoms of this disease are dry eyes, dry mouth, and fatigue. When initially diagnosed, individuals with Sjögren's may feel devastated due to the lack of curative treatment options, or they may feel a sense of satisfaction with finally knowing they have validation for the symptoms, especially knowing that it takes an average of 4.7 years to receive a proper diagnosis.[1] Regardless of how patients accept their official diagnosis, support groups and coping strategies should always be encouraged.

Patients with Sjögren's may struggle with psychological coping and physical health symptoms of the condition. Support groups aid in the process not only of coping with the symptoms but also helping to improve them. Many support groups encourage local doctors and specialists to attend to help educate patients and answer questions.

STRATEGIES FOR COPING

There are many strategies available to help cope with chronic diseases, such as Sjögren's. Coping can be defined as an individual's cognitive and behavioral efforts to manage stress.[2] In general, there are a variety of coping strategies for patients dealing with Sjögren's —some provide more favorable outcomes than others depending on

a Department of Oral Medicine, Carolinas Center for Oral Health, 1601 Abbey Place, Suite 220, Charlotte, NC 28209, USA; b Sjögren's Syndrome Foundation, 6707 Democracy Boulevard, Suite 325, Bethesda, MD 20817, USA; c Department of Oral Medicine, Carolinas Medical Center, 1000 Blythe Boulevard, Charlotte, NC 28203, USA
* Corresponding author.
E-mail address: Andrea.Herman@carolinashealthcare.org

Oral Maxillofacial Surg Clin N Am 26 (2014) 111–115
http://dx.doi.org/10.1016/j.coms.2013.09.011
1042-3699/14/$ – see front matter © 2014 Elsevier Inc. All rights reserved.

the patients. Some patients may enjoy personal interaction, whereas others may enjoy reading information. Many sources of coping mechanisms are available and patients should seek out what works best for their personal style.

TYPES OF COPING STRATEGIES
Emotion Focused

Emotion-focused coping strategies are targeted at reducing the distressful emotional reaction brought on by a situation. These strategies are an attempt to acknowledge, understand, and express emotions.[2] Patients' emotions can have an impact on their condition dramatically. If patients are more accepting of an incurable chronic condition, such as Sjögren's, their emotions could portray a positive outlook on the condition. By having a positive attitude, patients may not be as focused on the possible progression of their symptoms but instead on coping and treating the current ones. These positively focused patients may not concentrate on their symptoms every day.

Problem Focused

Problem-focused coping strategies involve active alterations of the person-environment relationship (ie, alterations of the source of stress). These strategies include both aggressive interpersonal efforts to alter a situation as well as rational, deliberate efforts to solve a problem.[2] Patients who have a negative outlook on the disease may automatically think their symptoms are getting worse and taking over their everyday life. These individuals stay extremely focused on the symptoms, especially the dry mouth and eyes. Sadness, depression, and decline in physical or social activity are common factors in patients that are emotionally impacted by Sjögren's in a negative way.

Avoidance

Avoiding the diagnosis or symptoms of Sjögren's can lead to many negative consequences. Avoidance coping includes strategies, such as denial and withdrawal.[2] Sjögren's patients can experience a wide range of symptoms ranging from dry mouth and eyes to neurologic problems to abnormal liver function to arthritis to gastrointestinal issues; being aware of active symptoms and other potential symptoms enables doctors to properly treat the patient. Avoidance of symptoms may lead to long-term damage of the body tissues, such as corneal damage from dry eyes and dental decay from dry mouth. Dry mouth (decreased saliva) can also lead to gastrointestinal problems, because there is not a sufficient amount of saliva to help break down food; thus, digestion can be interrupted.

ALTERNATIVE COPING STRATEGIES
Web-Based Coping

Social media is a phenomenal tool, allowing individuals from all over the world to instantly communicate about chronic conditions, such as Sjögren's. Credible Internet sources, such as the SSF Facebook page, the SSF blog located on www.sjogrens.org, Daily Strength: Sjögren's Syndrome Support Group, Sjögren's World, and MDJunction: Sjögren's Syndrome Support Group, can provide patients suffering from a chronic health condition with additional information about their illness, management options, and health improvement strategies. Patients should keep in mind, however, that information shared outside a credible source, such as the SSF, may be personal opinion and/or one person's experience with Sjögren's and may not translate to their personal circumstances. Patients always have to remember that knowledge is power; however, some information learned may not work for their particular case and/or may not be credible information at all. Appealing attributes of social media as a source for health-related information are low cost, convenience, and anonymous accessibility, allowing for 24-hour availability and providing updated, detailed information.[3] Media sources offer the ability to connect with others who have the disease while gaining support and knowledge from other patients.

Blogging communication enables people facing life challenges to simply and easily interconnect their progress with friends, family, and supporters and have those people respond with encouragement and help. It is a way to find others facing the same circumstances and exchange experiences and treatments within a safe online setting.[4] Also, patients can post their many struggles, accomplishments, and everyday thoughts to these Web sites to better cope with their issues. Blogs can assist patients with quick answers to their many questions concerning their disease.

Facebook is another way to establish a private social media group. Once a profile is established, an account can be set up as private so that only members can enter. The profile creator may then choose to accept other people into the group. Facebook is another way to interact with individuals privately so personal information about their experiences can be expressed.

Twitter is classified as instant messaging. It was created to share what someone is doing at any given moment with other people online. Twitter is a social networking tool for both business and personal uses. People who are coping with chronic disease can post broad questions or comments with little personal information.

Social Coping with Friends and Family

Close friends and family should be a main source of a patient's support system when dealing with a chronic illness. Social support may act as a shield, reducing the likelihood of undesirable life events from occurring, lessening the adverse impact of stressful events, or helping with the adjustment to a situation. Social support is classically conceived as a protective factor for health, whereas perceived social isolation is a major risk factor for morbidity and mortality.[5] It is important for patients' friends and family to understand what they are experiencing. Attending routine support group meetings with a friend or family member may provide insight to the patient's condition.

COPING WITH SJÖGREN'S SYNDROME

A study that compared stress, coping strategies, and social support in patients with primary Sjögren's found that most patients with primary Sjögren's experienced high psychological stress after major life events, prior to disease development. These patients did not successfully use coping strategies to confront their stressful life changes. The study concluded that lack of social support during times of psychological stress might contribute to the relative risk of disease development.[5]

Some researchers suggest that the perceived overall quality of life is the result of the impact of the disease-related symptoms (negative component) and the coping strategies used (positive component) to overcome the symptoms. The result of these two components determines the impact of the disease in everyday life.[6]

Because Sjögren's is a chronic condition, patients need to follow through with coping strategies throughout their lifetime. Patients should begin with seeking reliable information about their condition, try to manage symptoms of the syndrome daily, talk with others about the condition through local support groups or on the Internet, and take an active and positive role with the diagnosis. Patients can also try to use distractions, such as reading a book or playing a game, to take their minds off of the symptoms. Taking time to relax and thinking about the condition and the way it affects their life are essential and effective strategies for long-term coping. People suffering from Sjögren's may eventually feel encouraged knowing they are not alone with this chronic condition. Individuals may also seek spiritual or religious advice, become accepting of the disorder over time, and reinvest energy and knowledge into helping others.[7]

SUPPORT GROUPS FOR SJÖGREN'S SYNDROME

Support groups are used by patients with a wide variety of medical conditions and are sometimes distinguished from self-help groups by virtue of their professional or peer leadership.[8] These groups are known to bring individuals together with the same condition, such as rheumatoid arthritis, breast cancer, autism, and Sjögren's. For each support group, there is a different approach with that patient base. For example, a breast cancer group may want to focus on the discussion of breast reconstruction and raising money for research. An autism group may want to focus on early diagnosis in children whereas a rheumatoid arthritis group focuses on pain control of the joints. Sjögren's support groups tend to focus on treating current symptoms and discussing new treatment considerations along with ways to increase awareness of the disease.

The quality of life for patients with Sjögren's varies drastically. Some patients are primarily challenged with severe dental decay from their dry mouth or regular eye irritation from their dry eye. Others battle constant fatigue or joint pain but are still able to go to work while dealing with their illness whereas others are disabled, unable to work, and may apply for Social Security disability benefits. This disparity in how the disease affects each patient is why support groups are vital to helping all patients.

Pros and Cons with Support Groups

The pros for being involved in a support group for a disease or condition are
- There are other people with the same condition.
- Patients can bring family members to meet with the group to improve understanding of what the patients are experiencing.
- An individual can get ideas about alternative treatments and medications.
- A specialized doctor's contact information can be relayed to others.
- New products can be discussed to help treat symptoms.
- Breakthrough research can be announced to keep patients updated about the condition.

The cons for being involved in a support group for a disease or condition are

- Patients may hear about individual negative experiences with medications or treatments that may lead to them not trying a new and useful management strategy.
- The groups may only meet a couple times a year.
- If a group does not meet nearby, a patient may have to drive a long distance.

From these pros and cons, the authors believe that the benefits far outweigh the cons of a support group.

How a Support Group Functions

Patients or nonpatients can lead support groups. Support groups are commonly held 3 to 4 times per year, but more active groups meet more frequently. Patients are encouraged to attend with friends and family members, which brings others into their support network. These meetings are commonly held in the evening for approximately 1.5 hours. A strong network of Sjögren's syndrome support groups in the United States can be identified through the SSF. An individual may find information about the location of the groups on the SSF Web site and via mail announcements by the SSF.

The content of a support group meeting may include a wide range of topics, focusing on a particular symptom or be structured as a care-and-share format with no particular agenda. Meetings with a focused symptom for discussion may include a speaker, such as a rheumatologist, pharmacist, nutritionist, or dentist, who is familiar with a topic. The attendees are able to interact with the specialists in a group setting and individually, having access to ask specific, self-focused questions.

In a care-and-share type meeting, support group members have an opportunity to talk about their personal experiences on a wide range of topics related to Sjögren's, including struggles and triumphs. Patients also give insight into alternative treatments they have tried. In addition, they share their personal stories related to their diagnosis or support the family member of a newly diagnosed patient. Meetings can also be organized to include the combination of a structured topic in the first part of the meeting, followed by a discussion on general topics of interest for the members of the support group. At the end of most meetings, it is helpful to obtain suggestions on a specific topic for future gatherings (**Box 1**).

Box 1
How to form a support group

- Contact the SSF regarding assistance with communication with patients in the area. Join one of the SSF Support Group Leaders' educational conference calls.
- Establish a date, time, and venue (your home, local library, etc.) for the support group meeting, keeping in mind location, parking, accessibility and cost.
- Arrange an agenda with valid and interesting topics or a care-and-share focus. Be prepared to engage the attendees, keeping the meeting in line with the agenda.
- Schedule competent, knowledgeable speakers for the meeting (if applicable).
- Once an accurate number of potential attendees is received, purchase or obtain funding for light refreshments (if desired).
- During the meeting, ask for future meeting suggestions concerning speakers and topics.
- Plan the next support group to meet monthly, quarterly, or yearly.

Data from Brochures and resource sheets. 2011. Available at: http://www.sjogrens.org/home/about-sjogrens-syndrome/brochures-and-fact-sheets. Accessed May 31, 2013.

INFORMATION THROUGH SJÖGREN'S SYNDROME FOUNDATION

The SSF provides an extensive amount of credible information concerning Sjögren's. Obtaining accurate information concerning the disease at the time of diagnosis is crucial in allowing patients more control over a situation, enabling individuals to cope more positively with their progressing condition.[9] The SSF Web site provides information about the different symptoms and how they can affect life. Individuals can visit the Web site at www.sjogrens.org and view multiple categories for patients, health care providers, researchers, families and friends, donors, and members. The Web site also gives valuable information about the systemic disease, the foundation, research programs, member communities, awareness and diagnostic updates, new product information, and educational conferences.

The foundation also offers Sjögren's-related books, such as *The Sjögren's Syndrome Survival Guide* and *The Sjögren's Book* for purchase from the Web site. Individuals who become members of the SSF receive the monthly *Moisture Seekers* newsletter, which provides timely and informative question-and-answer sections, research updates, awareness campaign ideas, and coupons for specific products.

Sjögren's syndrome resource sheets are beneficial to doctors and patients. They are available online through the foundation. These sheets are 1-page summaries that focus on various symptoms of Sjögren's written by health care providers to include the following[10]:

- Airline travel tips: refers to Transportation Security Administration guidelines and travel tips
- Anti-inflammatory diet: foods that prevent inflammation and foods that cause inflammation
- Brain fog: what is brain fog and what can you do about it?
- Brittle nails tips: avoidances and protection for your nails
- Chronic pain tips: avoidances and recommendations for chronic pain
- Dental tips: suggestions to maintain the best oral health
- Disability benefits: obtaining disability benefits from the Social Security Administration
- Dry eye treatments: simple solutions for treating dry eye
- Dry nose and sinuses: simple solutions for dry nose and sinuses
- Dry skin: features and tips for dealing with dry skin
- Dry mouth treatments: simple solutions for treating dry mouth
- Fatigue fighters: techniques and coping strategies for fatigue
- Muscle and joint pain: recommendations and techniques to help with muscle and joint pain
- Oral candidiasis (thrush) in Sjögren's: avoidances and preventative measures for thrush
- Raynaud syndrome: suggestions to help control your Raynaud syndrome
- Reflux and your throat: tips for combating reflux in the throat
- Rheumatoid arthritis: the correlation between rheumatoid arthritis and Sjögren's syndrome
- Salivary glands massage: technique for massaging salivary glands
- Sex and Sjögren's: vaginal dryness, pelvic pain, fatigue, and mood symptoms
- Sleep tips: avoidances and recommendations for sleep
- Sun and Sjögren's: recommendations for ultraviolet radiation

- Surgery, hospitals, and medications: educating health care providers

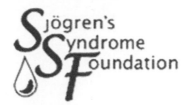

www.sjogrens.org

REFERENCES

1. Survey by the SSF and Polaris Marketing. 2013. Available at: http://info.sjogrens.org/conquering-sjogrens/bid/245451/Breaking-the-Barriers-4-7. Accessed June 13, 2013.
2. Roesch SC, Weiner B. A meta-analytic review of coping with illness: do causal attributions matter? J Psychosom Res 2001;50(4):205–19.
3. Van Uden-Kraan CF, Drossaert CH, Taal E, et al. Health-related Internet use by patients with somatic diseases: frequency of use and characteristics of users. Inform Health Soc Care 2009;34(1):18–29.
4. Living with dryness. Daily strength: Sjogren's syndrome support group. 2013. Available at: http://livingwithdryness.com/sjogrens-syndrome-support.php. Accessed May 31, 2013.
5. Karaiskos D, Mavragani CP, Makaroni S, et al. Stress, coping strategies and social support in patients with primary Sjogren's syndrome prior to disease onset: a retrospective case-control study. Ann Rheum Dis 2009;68(1):40–6.
6. Englbrecht M, Gossec L, DeLongis A, et al. The impact of coping strategies on mental and physical well-being on patients with rheumatoid arthritis. Semin Arthritis Rheum 2012;41(1):545–55.
7. Lauver DR, Connolly-Nelson K, Vang P. Stressors and coping strategies among female cancer survivors after treatments. Cancer Nurs 2007;30(2):101–11.
8. Finlayson ML, Cho CC. A profile of support group use and need among middle-aged and older adults with multiple sclerosis. J Gerontol Soc Work 2011;54(5):475–93.
9. Lode K, Larsen JP, Bru E, et al. Patient information and coping styles in multiple sclerosis. Mult Scler 2007;13(6):792–9.
10. Brochures and resource sheets. 2011. Available at: http://www.sjogrens.org/home/about-sjogrens-syndrome/brochures-and-fact-sheets. Accessed May 31, 2013.

Index

Note: Page numbers of article titles are in **boldface** type.

oralmaxsurgery.theclinics.com

Moving?

Make sure your subscription moves with you!

To notify us of your new address, find your **Clinics Account Number** (located on your mailing label above your name), and contact customer service at:

Email: journalscustomerservice-usa@elsevier.com

800-654-2452 (subscribers in the U.S. & Canada)
314-447-8871 (subscribers outside of the U.S. & Canada)

Fax number: 314-447-8029

Elsevier Health Sciences Division
Subscription Customer Service
3251 Riverport Lane
Maryland Heights, MO 63043

*To ensure uninterrupted delivery of your subscription,
please notify us at least 4 weeks in advance of move.

Moving?

Make sure your subscription moves with you!

To notify us of your new address, find your Clinics Account Number (located on your mailing label above your name), and contact customer service at:

Email: journalcustomerservice-usa@elsevier.com

800-654-2452 (subscribers in the U.S. & Canada)
314-447-8871 (subscribers outside of the U.S. & Canada)

Fax number: 314-447-8029

Elsevier Health Sciences Division
Subscription Customer Service
3251 Riverport Lane
Maryland Heights, MO 63043

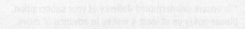

Printed and bound by CPI Group (UK) Ltd, Croydon, CR0 4YY

Printed and bound by CPI Group (UK) Ltd, Croydon, CR0 4YY

03/10/2024

01040378-0012